When Life Comes to a Standstill

WHEN LIFE COMES TO A STANDSTILL

The Surgeon Who Touches the Hearts of His Patients

Dr Ehsan Natour
Shirley Michaela Seul

Translated from the original German by Gert Reifarth, based on the book published by Scorpio Verlag München in February 2022, ISBN 978-3-95803-417-4. Co-author Shirley Michaela Seul.

English manuscript published by Dr Ehsan Natour. ISBN: 979-8-9862751-2-3 Hardcover, ISBN: 979-8-9862751-0-9 Paperback, ISBN: 979-8-9862751-1-6 eBook.

This book is not a medical textbook. The patient stories described here have been defamiliarized and transplanted into a fictional setting. The gender of the patients is of no importance, as one thing is indisputable; all human beings have a heart!

For those who entrusted their hearts to me.

And for you.

CONTENTS

In the same way as they prepare their children for other things in life such as school, love and jobs, I would like for every mother and every father to prepare their child for this:

One day, my son, my daughter, you will get into a situation which seems hopeless. It may seem to you that your life is ending. Or standing still. That might be because lovesickness prevents you from knowing how to continue to live, or because your business has to declare bankruptcy, or because your partner has died, or because you fail at something which is important to you. Or maybe you will receive a frightening diagnosis, or are deceived or abandoned. All this is part of life, and not a reason to think your fate is particularly hard. The longer you live, the higher the probability that you will encounter crises.

Approach these situations with trust. Free yourself from the expectation that you will afterwards be the same as before. Be open to the change and accept it; thus, you will manage it more easily. In this way you will not fight against things you cannot change, your fellow human beings will be better able to relate to you, your wounds will heal without complications. You will find a new normal more quickly if you don't try to hold on to the old one. What is normal in life is change. No normal is forever. And later, when you have survived the crisis – and you will, as you are well prepared – you will be better able to support others if their normal deserts them. Together, everything is easier, more beautiful and...healthier.

PROLOGUE

Where I come from, they say the soul lives in the heart and in the brain. During my training in Cologne, it was a shock for me when I saw an open chest without a heart for the first time. The patient was lying on the table, and there was a huge gaping hole where the heart should have been. But it was not there. The chief surgeon placed it in my hand while his assistant was preparing this patient's new heart. These two experienced colleagues performed a choreography which filled me with admiration. How confidently they balanced on the edge of death, virtually dancing on the green stage amongst all the shining stainless steel. How competently they made decisions that would decide the survival of the patient, who was deeply asleep, not noticing any of this. Or did he? Where did his soul sojourn? Definitely not in his heart, I realized in this moment, as I held it in my hand. Or was this no proof at all? It was a tired heart and had recently dragged itself through life with the utmost strain. It had become larger and larger and was eventually no longer able to support the patient's body properly. It appeared to me like an old person on their deathbed, and it spoke to me with a croaky and nearly broken voice: I can't go on.

Which is why it was replaced. With or without the soul? How many hearts is a person entitled to? And how does one live with a new heart or after any operation of similar severity? How does one live after a serious misfortune, when the old normal seems to have been cut from the body? Maybe it is simply a question of listening to the voice of one's heart. What would our world look like if we all did that?

These thoughts continue to concern me. Over the years, I have found answers to many of my questions, some of which I want to share with you in this book.

1

OPENING

I am about to open a thorax. Nothing is normal any more for the person in front of me on the operating table. I know this without talking to him. He would not be able to speak even if he wanted to, as he is lying in deep anesthesia in a dark green sterile landscape. The thorax area is all that is visible of him. But he no longer looks like he did on the beach where just yesterday he was cavorting with his two children...before IT happened, like a bolt from the blue, even though he is not yet forty years old. Youth does not protect you from illness.

The chest of this man who has become a patient overnight has been shaved and brushed all over with disinfectant. Rust orange meets dark green. Now here come my hands in beige-colored gloves. The scalpel flashes under the surgical lamp's strong light. Something incomprehensible is about to happen, something which has become second nature for me after thousands of operations. I will cut the skin with the scalpel, then open the sternum with the bone saw and reach deep inside him in order to save his life.

Now the heart is before me. A heart is more than an organ for me, it is like a living being. Each one is different. There are hearts which seem relieved when one is checking on them. Others appear depressed. There are sporty types and pudgy ones with too much fat. And very scared hearts like the one of these patients, whose heart told him to speak, as he told me before the operation: he was worried about his two children who are so close to his heart, and his wife whose heart would break if she were suddenly alone. We don't even notice how often we have our heart on our tongue; it is omnipresent as a symbol of love.

It was late when I sat at this patient's bed last night, but I knew he would not sleep. Pretty much nobody sleeps before a severe intervention. I always want to know who I'm operating on. In some clinics, surgeons only see the surgical area between the sterile green drapes. I want to know which human being the heart belongs to. That does not always work, as some heart operations are emergency procedures; more often than not the patients are unconscious when they are admitted. Other operations have been long planned: in six weeks, you will get a new heart valve, a bypass or whatever it may be. Everyone can prepare better for scheduled operations, including the patient's relatives. I prefer scheduled operations as they allow me to get to know my patients and their relatives, sometimes over several meetings. I know from my own experience – and many studies confirm it – that a good relationship between doctor and patient positively influences the healing process. Apart from this, I feel that the patients have a right to find out who will saw their sternum open, prod their heart, be by their side when their body is "dead", lying on a cooling blanket and cooled down to 25°C (77°F) – with a heart no longer beating, the heart-lung machine off and the aorta open. Only their brain is supported still, a small blood circuit keeps life going in the head while it has left the rest of the body. Will it return?

It still gives me goose bumps when a shut-down heart finds its way back to life – as if a musical composition were interrupted by a pause, the heart's music is silent for many bars of a movement, and then hopefully starts anew when the conductor raises his baton, which in this case is the wire of a defibrillator. In the operating room, too, the tension is palpable. Will the music of the heart sound again? Or are some instruments out of tune or, worse, forever silent? That, however, rarely occurs during an operation. What is critical is the time afterwards; this is not known to many patients who believe that the worst is behind them once they have survived the operation.

If you have read until this point, reader, you are brave – and wise. Some people only deal with a problem once they're up to their neck in it. By reading this book, you are preparing yourself for the unknown. It does not have to be heart surgery, but any of the risk's life has in store for us all. Maybe you are facing a crisis right now; in some way, we are all in crisis mode ever since COVID-19 first emerged. We hope for everything to become normal again as quickly as possible. We become only gradually aware that there is no normal we are entitled to – that this insistence on a normal even weighs down on our lives considerably. There is a better and much healthier way, namely, to flexibly adjust to the challenges. We will go a stretch of this road together in this book. At the end you may share my opinion that our healthcare system needs a few major interventions in order to keep an eye not merely on a person's body but also on their quality of life. Even though we may function perfectly as performers in a performance society, no one is immune against the occasional aches and pains, accidents, illnesses, and unforeseen events.

How do we approach people who have fallen out of our unspoiled, well-functioning mainstream? This includes those who are healthy but still at their wits' end – because their professional existence has been destroyed or someone close to them has fallen seriously ill. An illness, after all, does not only befall one person. Like a bomb it can shatter a vast social landscape. Will we avoid those affected because we don't know how to behave around them? The older we become, the more likely it is that we are relatives and friends of people who have to cope with serious misfortune, who may need a partner with whom they can discuss the most intimate things. Ideally, they will endure this crisis – because they do not run away but are prepared to deal with it, and because they do not insist on a normal long gone but adjust bravely and flexibly to their new situation. If they are successful, things are easier for everyone.

But of course, it is tempting to pretend to be one's "old self" again, because which "new self" should one be? It is yet unknown and therefore frightens us. What we do not know is frightening to us and we reject it initially. If a society as a whole is primarily interested in smooth proceedings and in the quick restoration of people's smooth functionality after an illness, we have no blueprint for how matters could be different. To function means to play one's roles. The husband must go back to his role as "family executive", the boss must go back to his business, grandma looks after everyone, this person always cracks a joke, that person continues to play the strong one who gets everything done...and what does the heart have to say about this, our inner voice?

Go slowly.
Is this really important?
Is this good for you?
What do you need right now?

Your only chance of conquering fear is to talk about it. Fear divides. Trust and love connect. Whoever talks about fear diminishes it. But we must practice that. As human beings, and as doctors, too.

Some doctors have a fear of speaking with patients; this occurs more often than one would think. After all, who would want to tell a person that they don't have much longer to live? In my experience, the better way in such situations, too, is to connect with a patient rather than to remain separated from them, for example by using medical jargon or outsourcing: "Dear colleague, would you explain the diagnosis to the patient."

Sometimes a colleague asks me why I "bother" with the personal contact to my patients when I could make it much easier for myself. Cut open, repair, sew up – and anything further will be dealt with in intensive care. To operate conveyor-belt style is everyday practice in big hospitals. You start with operation one and work your way through to operation four, and all you see is bodies covered with green drapes. The hole in the drapes is where my job begins.

In the intensive care units of our high-performance medicine, playing God is quite common – and not always with the patients' wellbeing in mind. Hardly anything seems impossible. There is no such thing as "can't be done". We can do anything. Thus, heart medicine turns patients into cases, and the human beings within the patients into defects which have to be repaired. As a result of this fixation on feasibility, even the joy in it, some people sadly overlook the fact that there is not only an illness, but also an ill person – who needs something very old-fashioned, namely love and care and time to gather strength again and get well. Our modern medicine takes its cue from the natural sciences, and more and more from profitability. Hospitals should be in the black, patients are administrated, and before patients have even spoken with a doctor, lump-sum payments dictate the duration of their recovery and the length of their stay in hospital. Medical staff have to devote a lot of time and attention to case documentation; this time is taken away from their contact with patients. Instead of such personal contact, we can observe that consultations are replaced by machines and measurements. The sick human becomes a faulty workpiece which has to be repaired in a predetermined amount of time. And that is exactly how some patients feel. I have even observed a further escalation: more and more patients do not even expect for a doctor to be seriously interested in them, to really listen to them. They are surprised when they are examined instead of just connected to machines. Ordinarily, it is a little like a car repair shop where we rarely find mechanics with oily hands anymore but rather diagnostic computers.

I notice this when patients become quite unsettled by

the smallest act of love and care, or when they remark that a doctor touched them: "Imagine, he examined me, really examined me. With his hands."

Touch is a primary, fundamental human experience. Even before a newborn sees or sucks, they are touched, held tenderly by their parents. With touch, our organism releases numerous hormones including the so-called cuddle hormone oxytocin. We feel meaningful, secure, appreciated.

In a section called "What makes my life richer" of the German weekly paper *Die Zeit*, at Easter 2020, I read of a small gesture which had been made by a white coat towards a patient. The patient thought it so unusual that she sent an account of it to the paper, and the editors in turn deemed it so remarkable that they published the piece.

I had to undergo an operation of the gall bladder, a delicate affair. "How are you?", asked the senior doctor during the first ward round after the surgery. "Any bowel movement yet?" Me: "With this weak coffee there is no chance of any bowel movement." He replied: "I know what you mean. You need a nice black coffee, and I will get you one..." And indeed, after the round he came back to my room with a double espresso.[1]

A surgeon does not necessarily have to speak to their patients to do a good job. But I believe that it makes things easier for the patients if they get to know their surgeon. I also regard contact with the patients a fulfillment of my profession. This may be due to the course of my career development. Born in the border area between Palestine and Israel and growing up Arabic-Israeli as someone who had to negotiate that border, I now work at the border between life and death. I like people, like to be together with lots of them – not surprising with ten siblings and a very large family. I like things to be…intense!

The White Snake

After finishing high school in Israel, I moved to Germany where two of my brothers were already studying – without the university fees so common in many other countries. Otherwise, my family could not have afforded the education of so many children eager for knowledge. Today we have a film producer, a school principal, two school secretaries, two directors of social institutions, two engineers, two doctors and one professor in my family. My first port of call in Germany was Heidelberg. After a year at a language school, I studied medicine in Kiel. This time formed me, as I was earning my living as an assistant nurse, and probably also set my inner clock: since then, I have been used to night shifts – which were the best-paid shifts back then, so that I would secure at least one night shift per week on top of the normal ones. Which was why my course took me a year longer to complete than other students…a person needs some time to sleep after all. When I think back today, I know that many of my experiences in Kiel's neurosurgery unit shaped my attitude to colleagues as well as patients. I learned things from scratch. We assistant nurses made beds, washed and fed patients, administered medication, and frequently we (together with the nurses) were the only audience for the things which afflicted the souls of the patients, which would often weigh them down more than physical pain. Often, we would translate what the doctors had meant, and explain the jargon. Many years were still to pass until I was in a position myself to turn to the complete patient and see them as a whole being, both physically and psychologically.

After my studies, I spent an eighteen-month internship as a doctor in Cologne. I had already abandoned the plan to become a neurosurgeon – surgery yes, but brain no thank you, as interesting as my years in Kiel had been. In Cologne I was part of the ward rounds, even though I was far back in the queue of medics snaking into patients' rooms. The affair was just as patient-unfriendly as it had been in Kiel – when indeed the ward round is the highlight of the day for the patients. The professor is approaching! Or the senior physician! In their sleepless nights, the patients prepare themselves, search for the right phrases to best put into words their burning issues, and how to make it quick as one knows the white coats are always pressed for time and one does not want to slow them down or inconvenience them.

Come with me to a patients' room with three people in it. One is lying next to the window, looking out. *Up in that tree there's a blackbird, oh how I wish I was outside.* The patient in the middle is sitting on her bed, packed suitcases on her mind. When will she be allowed to go home? She's been here for three weeks, after all. Close to the door, the third patient has pulled her blanket up to her chin, feeling cold, nevertheless. Simultaneously with a knock the door flies open, and the medics making the rounds sweep in at 7.37am. What the patients don't know is that there is a ward conference scheduled for 8 o'clock – but the "white snake" following the senior physician knows. Not even thirty minutes for thirty patients. And even though the three in this room have been waiting for the ward round for hours, they are now overwhelmed and much too slow to follow the frantic pace. With an effort, the patient at the window who would like to swap places with the blackbird starts to turn around. There is no space for all the white coats, only the snake's head, while the rest remains in the corridor and misses the ward round – just like the woman at the window, because before she has managed to face the door, the white snake is already on its way to the next room.

"What did he say", a young medic murmurs to an assistant doctor.

"Mrs. Meier, three bypasses yesterday, all going well."

"And the others?"

"Everything's normal."

"But I wanted to ask if I can go home", the patient in the middle bed will later tell the nurse in a worried tone. The whole night she had concocted her sentence, pondering whether she should mention her grandchild or her caring husband to try and speed up her release. But there had been no time, no time for anything. Now she will have to wait until tomorrow, even though she had been well prepared as she had already showered, brushed her teeth and done her hair so that the senior doctor would see how fit she is. But he did not even see her. Everything's normal.

By now I have worked in hospitals for decades, and things have not improved there since my time as an assistant nurse – on the contrary. It does not help patients to be seen merely as a bypass or a gall bladder or a carcinoma. There are human beings attached to the illnesses, and if I see that human being, I gain a different insight into the situation. I am not a psychologist, but I wonder why we should try to further improve a system in which both sides are not doing so well: not only the patients suffer under the circumstances, but also the doctors. Everything nowadays has become even faster than back then – everywhere, not just in hospitals. Time seems to accelerate more and more, and everyone is stressed. In everyday hospital life you feel downright hunted sometimes, and yet white snakes on ward rounds continue to rush from one room to the next – when it would maybe take just one minute to say "Good morning" and have a look at the wound. A few small things will make the patients feel they are in good hands. Their pulse will slow down, and they relax, which is exactly what they need to recover and get well again.

And isn't this just what many doctors want as well? Sometimes I ask myself why we so often forget that we are human beings with human needs – all of us, no matter which side we are on. One group wants to get well, the other wants to make them well. We know what is conducive to our health and what is not…stress, for example, and yet stress is growing and growing. What is really dangerous here is that we get used to it, becoming unable to find a way out of a crisis. We are going round in circles, constantly increasing the speed with which we enter a dead-end street.

Many people who are attracted by medicine as a profession feel a high level of inner motivation. Nurses told me countless times that they entered this profession because it is meaningful for them, and they can do something good and improve things. Unfortunately, they realize after only a short time that the system in which they work does not support their motivation or even destroys it. This frightening conclusion has not yet penetrated wider society, as otherwise we would hardly wonder about the dwindling numbers of the nursing staff we so badly need.

A solution would be to focus on a phenomenon mentioned by many people whose motivation remains high: I get back more than I give. It is true – even in the direst situation people who depend on help from others still have something to give. This touches me greatly, and I know many such moments. They are one reason for writing this book: I want to pass on things which my patients have taught me…and thereby make it easier for those who have the path through a crisis still before them.

At least these days I – now at the head of the "white snake" – can do things differently, even though I know that in many clinics there is no "Good morning" to this day, let alone thirty "Good mornings" or "Goodbyes". The time that would waste when everyone knows time is money!

But is that true? Is it not rather the case that at the end of the day one saves money with "Good Mornings" and "Goodbyes" as the patients feel well looked after? When you talk with someone you get to know each other, and this may well lead to a better diagnosis. In my opinion, good communication is one of the most important tasks of a doctor – but it is the most difficult one for many. Some young health professionals are not even aware of the fact that good contact with their patients is an essential tool of their profession. That is despite our knowledge from psychoneuroimmunology (which examines the interdependence between body and soul) as to how important trust is for the stimulation of our self-healing powers: mental processes directly affect our immune system and thus shape our resistance against infectious diseases and positively influence the healing of wounds. The more relaxed patients are, and the better they feel, and the more trust they have in their medical environment, the greater are their chances of healing. I believe that a "Good morning" on a ward round, followed by a "How are you?" is the absolute minimum. And one should touch each patient at least once, briefly place a hand on their body. This alone calms the patient down, as numerous studies show. *I'm looking out for you. I'm looking after you. You are in good hands.*

Back to my career. I wanted to become just such a doctor and never lost this ideal in all my further ports of call, which at times led to a little trouble for me but also lots of appreciation. After a few years in Cologne, I moved on to Oldenburg, now as a senior doctor and specialist for heart surgery. In Oldenburg we operated on many people who got an artificial heart while they were waiting for an organ donation. I also became a specialist for vascular surgery. The aorta starts at the heart and reaches down to the groin, and to replace it is a lengthy matter – my longest operation took twenty-six hours.

When I became a father for the second time, I moved to a clinic in Groningen because working conditions are more humane in the Netherlands than they are in Germany. In my opinion, the German health system can learn a lot from the Dutch one – for the benefit of patients and doctors alike. In the Netherlands, quality of life is much more prominent, and we ask if this or that procedure will improve it. In Germany, feasibility is more important, prompting intensive care units not infrequently to take superfluous measures which not only put a strain on patients but can even harm them.[2]

A study at a German university clinic showed that every tenth cancer patient was reanimated in an ICU during the last week of their lives. Is this a gain in quality of life, or rather a prolonging of suffering? The same is true for patients with severe dementia who are admitted into ICUs and given artificial respiration – without any positive effect for them. I would like to see us emphasize the question of the quality of life rather than that of feasibility, as feasibility is often the cause of cruel ordeals – which is true also for life outside hospitals.

In Groningen I was a member of a heart-and-lung transplantation team. I shut down the still-beating hearts of brain-dead patients, extracted them and implanted them into other patients. After eight years my path led me to Maastricht and Aachen, and today I operate in both cities.

From the beginning I was interested in how people's lives would continue after surgery. Normally the surgeon does not find out about this, as the different departments are separated from each other. In my opinion we should connect them. We can only learn if we find out how things continue "afterwards".

What does life look like after an operation, how do people handle a second chance? In my experience it is not a good path to return to normality as quickly as possible – and it does not work anyway. If we put ourselves under pressure for everything to return to what it was, we miss a great chance and, in the case of illness, maybe even life. This insight applies to crises as well as illnesses. But we live in a time where the impossible is to be possible, and at all times. After all, we are so sophisticated! We explore space, we transplant more than one organ at the same time... but what about ourselves? Within the limits of our bodies? Is the notion of "being top-notch" of importance here? When something happens that makes us say:

"My heart just stopped."

This book balances on the razor's edge of situations when life seems to stand still. Hearts don't stand still only during heart surgery, but they are in a state of shock also during a car crash, an outbreak of cancer or a life crisis… and we say so, too: "My heart just stopped." *My heart stopped* – I still exist elsewhere but something in me has stopped.

Sometimes, however, *everything* stops. For a few seconds, minutes, or a longer time. It is as if one enters a space void of air, a vacuum. And in this vacuum, questions arise.

How do you measure the quality of life?

Do we have the right to health?

How can we, as a society, deal with the fear of illness and uncertainty?

And as an individual?

How much am I worth if I can't perform like I used to?

Who am I if I identify with my illness?

And if I don't?

What can I learn from a crisis?

And when should we stop fighting death?

A Matter of the Heart

An intense medical treatment affects not only the patients and their environment but everyone who is connected with it, including the doctors and nursing staff. Emotions far beyond the scope of the normal are triggered in everyone who is involved, especially when a heart is shut down. That's why it is so important to analyze these emotions and grant them appropriate space, to prevent them from being ignored and potentially causing harm at the wrong moment. Processing them properly prepares you for a good life afterwards.

For many years now I have explored how people deal with diagnoses, which behavior is beneficial and which is harmful – and I have reached interesting conclusions which have not yet been put into practice in current medicine. Maybe that will change once we publish the results of our study. At our clinic in Maastricht, we have investigated since 2020 how anxiety impacts the healing process. We classify the patients into different categories and offer them tailor-made therapy – personalized medicine. Anxious patients require a different therapy than those who are emotionally stable. The better the patients prepare for the operation and particularly the time afterwards, the more they will be able to reclaim their quality of life. Most importantly, they will have understood that it is not only the operation that matters, but that the time afterwards is significant as well. Most people think no further than their operation – once it's done, I will be over the hump. That is a fatal error. The operation may set the course for a new life, but for it to gather steam depends on the patient and on the specific circumstances, the environment. When we fall ill, it is not only our own life that changes. An illness also has repercussions for our environment, which in turn affects our perception of ourselves – everything is connected. Therefore, it is a mistake to believe that one can view and treat illnesses in isolation.

I am very happy to have found fellow comrades in arms for the matter closest to my heart which first came to light nearly twenty years ago. The *Stilgezet* foundation was born in the Netherlands in 2019 to promote the topic internationally. *Stilgezet* is a Dutch word which describes a temporary standstill caused by a medical diagnosis or a life crisis.

After the foundation, this book is our second step, and many more will follow – not only theoretical, medical ones, but artistic ones most prominently. Art, after all, enables us to describe many things for which science lacks the means of expression. The arts can name the unsayable, find images for it and transpose them into music, for example. Love and death, fear, rage, sadness, helplessness – none of this can be operated away by a heart surgeon. Art can lead us to insights which help us process our experiences and make us realize that we are not alone. Artistic expression can also help us cope with a new normal.

I gained this insight at the Christmas market in Oldenburg. Even today I can see myself standing next to a fire basket near a stall that sold candied almonds, looking into the flames. I was not in a good mood, as my mind had become caught up in thoughts about a specific patient. I did not recognize myself like this – haunted by someone's fate. I was annoyed with it and with me. Was it really the right thing to do, to let my patients touch me this closely? Then again, they let me come close to them, too: it is giving and taking. Connection needs closeness.

The aorta of a thirty-year old man had ruptured in a car accident. His chances of survival were very poor, particularly since he had been given blood thinners during emergency treatment, which make sewing nearly impossible as the tissue becomes like butter. He was conscious when I met him.

"Please help me", he pleaded. To understand him I

leaned over him, placing my ear to his mouth. "I have three small children."

Three small children? They affected me, settled firmly in my heart. I am a father myself after all. Did that make me lose the professional distance which normally kicked in automatically? This distance does not have to be cold – I can be caring and affectionate and still professional. I had operated on many fathers before. Then why had this patient been cruising through my mind for days? The operation had been successful, but he had died in intensive care. Three children had lost their father. It was them I was thinking of when I looked into the fire.

Suddenly someone spoke to me, "Hello Doc." I turned to the nurse who like me was strolling through the Christmas market near the hospital. He was a little older than me and very experienced. We liked each other. He held his bag of fragrant almonds towards me invitingly while we exchanged a few words. Then he asked me directly: "What's up with you?"

"What do you mean?", a reflex made me return the question, while it hit me in that moment how deeply the loss of this patient had affected me.

"You seem heavy-hearted", the nurse said. "That is quite striking with someone whose nature – fitting with his name – is usually so cheerful", he smiled.

I felt the spontaneous urge to protest. Why, what should be up with me, I was okay, wasn't I? I took the time to listen to my inner voice – to my heart, one could say. The nurse did not say anything, just stood beside me. We looked into the fire in silence for a while. Then I told him about my patient. He listened attentively and, in the end, said something I will never forget: "You don't have to be sad, something like that is not in your hands. It is in the hands of God. He sent this patient to you."

From this moment, I never again toyed with the idea of locking my own heart in order to save lives with a cool head. I understood that I could do that with a feeling heart, too. I sought an active connection, like the heart-lung machine during an operation. My connection started before the operation and did not end when the hearts of my patients were beating again. To what rhythm were they beating? I was interested in their new heart music, in their whole postoperative life, and I realized that the processes in play here were not restricted to heart surgery but applied to any operation, any illness, any crisis. I saw every day how much better patients were managing if they were well prepared and had known from the beginning that the old normal would cease to exist, and that it may take much longer than expected before they will have adjusted to their new life. Thinking all this through helped reduce their fear. Ideally, they were curious about the new normal, which in turn would merely be a new stage on their life's path. Some of my patients indeed find life more beautiful now, even though it is more restricted. They feel it more intensely, they have become aware of its value – which is what matters. And I, too, felt different since that evening on the Christmas market. A fire was flaring inside me.

The matter closest to my heart was born. And now it would be lovely if I could reach your heart, too.

[1] Source: *Die Zeit*. Marianne Link from Altötting, Bavaria.

[2] https://link.springer.com/article/10.1007/ s00740-019-0288-8.

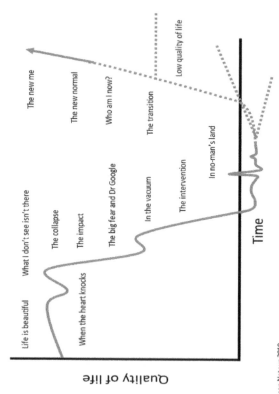

2

LIFE IS
BEAUTIFUL

When did you last notice that life is beautiful? Just like that: *life is beautiful*. Isn't it crazy that we often appreciate life merely in retrospect when it is on the verge of withering? When it is threatened? Is this maybe a feature of a beautiful life – that we do not realize how beautiful it is? Ideally, that is the normal state of affairs, which is why we do not think about it, or only if we come into contact with people or news which show that life is not beautiful for everyone.

Of course, there are days when our life, too, may not run so perfectly. For instance, if a visit to the dentist is coming up...but the day after tomorrow all will be well again, and then it will go on like that, on and on – given one ranks among the optimists. Now and then the thought may surface that something awful may happen, but we brush that aside quickly. Now and then something awful may happen which in retrospect – when something *really* awful has occurred – we deem not so awful any longer: "It was only a small matter. How could I get so upset about it?" Well, if today we are in a crisis, we deem life back then beautiful. But did we perceive it like that back then? Did we live in the Now?

Beautiful life takes place in the moment. I noticed that a few years ago when I automatically reached for my cellphone when I woke up. I fed yesterday's news to the person I am today. I was also busy thinking about the future, namely the operation which was ahead of me. But where was the present? Was it the fact that I would enjoy a wonderful coffee at home on this early morning...well, in ten minutes, I had raced ahead again? But then, coffee cup in hand, I was able to enjoy the moment, which was so beautiful I added a few more to it.

Since then, I have abstained from looking at yesterday's news in the mornings – a diet I can recommend! In the mornings I reward myself with some free space, some emptiness in which the new day can unfold. That feels good, because once the day starts to run (and most of my days go at high speed), I can no longer find quiet time. Sure, I could remind myself that life is beautiful when I am looking into an open thorax. I love my job. But honestly, in a situation like that I have other thoughts on my mind, for example about how soon will we be able to stop a patient's bleeding.

At some stage, bleeding will occur somewhere in the system of beautiful life, too. That is normal, part of being human. Just a little tear, a little injury which the body can repair quickly. The body is a master of healing everything. But we are unaware of this highly complex process, even though many different cells are involved as well as neurotransmitters and other substances which work together to repair a defective area as quickly as possible. They all act in concert. The most important thing is to stop the bleeding, which is of course minimal with such a small tear, not like during a heart surgery when blood might spurt up to the lamp.

Hemostasis is achieved by vasoconstriction and the activation of blood coagulation. After a small injury, inflammation is triggered to increase the permeability of the small blood vessels. This creates more blood plasma, a secretion which cleans the wound. Foreign matter, cell debris and bacteria are flooded out. White blood cells help in the role of phagocytes. In the next step, after a few days a network of new tissue begins to grow into the injured area. Stabilizing protein fibers pull the edges of the wound inward so that the wound shrinks. At the end of the healing process comes the phase of regeneration which can last several weeks depending on the size of the wound.

Scars remain. Every one of us has suffered some, on the inside and on the outside. We may even be proud on some of them, while we have forgotten others. The body, however, forgets nothing – but it knows that we like to forget certain things, which is why it reminds us of them sometimes: it may knock on our door with some pain, or a limitation which we deem annoying. It can also knock with a suspicion: was it really a girlfriend your wife was at the movies with? Or a worry: will the client pay the bill? In the same way our body issues warnings, we often receive them in life. Hardly anything happens out of the blue. If we think about it later, once lightning has struck us, we notice that there had been hints. We did not see or hear them, because we did not want to hear or see them – because we want everything to remain how it is.

It is because of this desire that we ignore the voice of our heart. It knocks, again and again, but we have no time. The body compensates over and over, repairing blood vessels, healing wounds, relaxing tense muscles – all these things are the results of highly complex processes which take place without us noticing them. Maybe we will feel a little groggy for a day: "I'm not at my best today." Our immune system may be battling with an army of attackers. On the next day things will be better again. Even if not, we'll just plow on as always, because that is the normal thing to do, and we don't have time for any kind of drama. Sure thing – who the hell fancies a catastrophe? But that attitude won't prevent it. Did it not grant us enough chances, again and again? We will only notice that later, if at all. Hindsight is easier than foresight.

One knows that beforehand, but it's no use – as we heard from politicians who explained during the pandemic: "We will know later if we did the right thing." A pandemic, however, does not knock in the same way a first suspicion does, or a disturbance of well-being, or a strange feeling that something is wrong. If we speak of a pandemic, it is too late. COVID-19 did not have to catch us unprepared. There had been warning voices which pointed to an imbalance in the relationship between humans and nature. But they weren't heard because listening to them would have meant leaving our comfort zone. And wasn't everything running smoothly? No, things had not run smoothly for a long time. Life's rhythm had been disturbed.

When the Heart Knocks

Normally, the heart beats sixty to eighty times per minute. It carries nine thousand liters of blood daily, beating about one hundred thousand times in the process. It has been doing this job from day twenty-two after your conception.

So, your heart is, in a manner of speaking, older than you are – after all, you presumably do not remember the moment of your first heartbeat. Ever since then, your heart has been beating and beating and beating, mostly unnoticed. Most people prefer it like that; they believe that not noticing their heart means everything is fine. If suddenly we *do* notice something, when our heart loses its rhythm without any obvious explanation like exercise or agitation or love, we are alarmed. The heart is allowed to skip a beat, it is even normal, for example when we go for a jog, so our heart beats faster, or we are in love and our heart becomes a butterfly fluttering in our stomach, or there was a near miss when a truck took our right of way and our heart is in our mouth. But when the heart stumbles without any obvious reason, depending on our personality, we visit a doctor immediately or ignore the matter until it knocks on our door again.

Arrhythmia can indeed be within the realm of the normal – it is merely an extrasystole. The term "systole" refers the contraction of the myocardium during the expectoration of blood from the ventricles into our circulation. An extrasystole means the heart is doing an extra shift, maybe because we are stressed or overtired or have high blood pressure at the moment. A cardiac cycle consists of a contraction phase (called systole) and a relaxation phase (called diastole) during which the ventricles fill up with blood again. If the heart stumbles just a little, we won't realize it. Serious extrasystoles, however, we will notice as they interrupt our normal rhythm. Other events in our life, too, may disturb that rhythm. How do we deal with it, knowing deep down that it doesn't come without a reason? Do we listen to the voice of our heart? How often will it have to knock before we are willing to recognize that something's going on that we should take care of?

The more closely we listen, the better; because waiting too long can turn a small inconvenience into a big drama, a slight misunderstanding may turn into a catastrophe.

Life *Has* to Be Beautiful: What I Don't See Isn't There

"Ah forget it! Nothing's wrong!" A small voice may whisper: "But something *is* wrong." Yet we don't want to listen to that, because life is beautiful, and it is to remain so. And remain it does – until the next irritation arrives. Much time may pass until then, or only a few days, hours, minutes – like with a heart attack. Crises are polite, as mentioned above they usually make themselves known by knocking, which will cause our hearts to beat. We hold on to what we have as we are afraid of losing it, intuitively sensing that the situation may be dangerous. "Don't single us out, dear God, make everything well again. My wife and I have a good marriage. I've done everything…" This betrays our fear and shows how much we resist the facts and instead ignore them as imaginary.

No, not me. It's just a knock. Everything may turn out well still, which means it will remain as it is. Life is beautiful, and a little palpitation does not mean anything.

When the heart beats fast because of stress or fear, it is nothing but a mechanism of compensation. It beats faster because it always pumps the same amount of blood in the same amount of time. But when the vessels widen (as happens when we feel stress or fear), the heart must pump more blood and does so by increasing either intensity or speed. When we engage in physical exercise, too, the pulse increases to ensure that feet and head receive the necessary amount of blood. But there are other reasons for an increased heartbeat such as a narrowing heart valve which creates resistance the heart has to overcome. Over time, this will affect the myocardium, which will become thicker and thicker...what would be a joy for any bodybuilder is not healthy for the heart. This physical reaction may lead to a crisis. To bring down the pulse, beta-blockers are required or possibly a new valve.

In the case of a calcified valve, shortness of breath is a main symptom. One goes up the stairs and has difficulty breathing. I should exercise again, one may think, and does not do it – because one has difficulty breathing. Lack of air is not always due to bad fitness. Apart from a defective valve, it can have other causes – which are now knocking. But we do not want to hear them, not see them, wishing to remain in our normal. We know all about that. That's where we're safe, that's where we believe all is well – when in reality something awful is brewing.

Six months or sometimes up to two years after an operation, an enlarged heart will be back to its normal size. Back to the old normal? No – it is beating in its *new* normal. The sooner a patient listens to the first error messages and the cries for help from his heart and body, the less complicated it will be for their new normal to shape itself.

If you think back: wasn't it true that nothing happened after the first hint, it took a second one...which hits the mark. We delay our bankruptcy; how much easier would it have been to react immediately. A dead relationship is continued over years; how liberating would it have been to break up. Many patients understand only after their second hospitalization that things are serious. Or how serious. Skin cancer. You should not go out into the sun anymore. Yes, but the summer's so lovely. Diet is another topic we like to brush aside: one knows one should eat more healthily, but the other stuff tastes so good.

Oh well, it'll be fine.

But when the heart is involved, looking away can be life-threatening, as one day all compensation mechanisms will fail. The body can no longer balance the bad things a person subjects it to. A relationship can no longer withstand all the cheating, a job can no longer endure the bullying, a bank account is now permanently in the red…whatever it may be. It was okay for a while, even though the motor was no longer running on all four cylinders. In the end, only one or two were left, and the breakdown can no longer be avoided.

When one's health is concerned, the second warning may be the last, for example when it is a heart attack. For many, that is an awful prospect – even though they have no idea how the heart works. That is in fact symptomatic – we don't deal with it, hoping it will be alright. Yet we can only react properly if we prepare for whatever may happen. So, I will include a little account of how the heart works here. Don't worry, one paragraph will be enough.

The fist-sized myocardium provides vital oxygen and nutrients by pumping between two and twenty liters of blood through the body every minute. This enormous effort is carried out by two ventricles (right and left atrium) and two main chambers (right and left ventricle).

The heart pumps blood rich in oxygen via the main artery (the aorta) into other arteries which branch out into ever smaller blood vessels (the capillaries). Then the blood low in oxygen flows from the tissue back to the heart through the veins. Aorta means fresh blood; veins mean old blood. Back in the heart, the blood is pumped into the pulmonary circulation and is enriched with oxygen once again. Our cardiovascular system starts another cycle. A heart which is alive is rooted deeply in the body, and its blood vessels are connected with every single one of our many billion cells. Its pathways reach deep into us and far up to our brain, with millions of branches which become finer and finer. Heart surgeon and author Reinhard Friedl, in his book *The Beat of Life*, even calls the heart our most important sensory organ. Four valves regulate our blood circulation. Like mechanical valves, they make sure that the blood can only flow in one direction. The so-called sinus node sets the rhythm – which occasionally loses its beat.

3

THE COLLAPSE

A heart attack does not knock politely, it crashes through the door – and brutally. Occasionally it can also sneak up on you quietly as a so-called silent heart attack which will later come to light as an accidental diagnosis. As a rule, however, a heart attack is a classic case of code red. Without thinking about it, we place a hand on our chest when we get a fright or hear bad news.

A "normal" heart attack is accompanied by strong pain in the chest area, called angina pectoris, which spreads to arms, back, abdomen or neck. Suddenly, patients feel not just weak but completely without strength. They are pale, sweating and usually know with terrible certainty that something life-threatening is occurring to them. Strong men, too, no longer wave it aside thinking it will be okay, but pant in a strained voice: "Call an ambulance." And that is the right decision, because a heart attack means that an artery is acutely occluded.

Panic sets in, fear of death – which is completely justified. The patients know that they need help immediately. Will I make it to the phone? Which number? They sense that unconsciousness is a threat. They are completely alone; their fight for life holds them in its grip, and sometimes they will not escape it. Numerous patients experience arrhythmia in such an acute crisis; they become unconscious as a result and are only found hours or days later. Their heart is silent... forever.

Many people think that heart attacks are a male phenomenon. That is incorrect, but the number of heart attacks in females is dwarfed by male ones as the latter occur earlier and men are often torn from their "best years" by a heart attack while they are still working. The heart attack of a female pensioner is not as spectacular as when the chairman suddenly puts a hand to his chest in the middle of a board meeting, contorts his face and collapses. That is how they like to show it in movies, and nowadays it is part of general knowledge that tightness in the chest and pain in the left arm point to a heart attack. With women, there are additional and different symptoms, which makes their heart attack so dangerous for them: malaise, nausea, shortness of breath – "have I upset my stomach?" This wrong track may cost a life because too much time is lost before the heart attack is diagnosed.

But what exactly is a heart attack? "The pump is on strike", a patient once very appropriately described this acute artery occlusion, as a result of which the myocardium dies off, which in turn causes arrhythmia. And there is a long process preceding this, even though the heart attack appears to happen suddenly. The risk factors are known high cholesterol, high blood pressure, smoking, alcohol, obesity, diabetes, lack of exercise, stress. All this leads to arteriosclerosis. Colloquially, the sediments in the arteries are called calcification; doctors use the term plaque.

The body compensates for the calcification for a long time. Once a vessel is decisively narrowed, other smaller vessels take over its function. They can enlarge themselves considerably to meet the new tasks. I call them "buddy" vessels. One does not abandon one's buddy, and together they do everything to keep the big buddy – the person – alive. But a small buddy by itself cannot manage to take over the tasks of a big vessel. Therefore decompensation occurs at a certain point in time, as the detour path becomes overloaded – and a heart attack is the consequence. Before that happens, when the mechanisms of compensation start to fail, there can also be unconsciousness and shortness of breath. A person may take this seriously or else pretends that nothing happened – it is a decision which can determine for how long he or she will remain on this beautiful planet.

Specialists Save Lives
Many people believe that heart surgeons and cardiologists are the same thing. However, cardiologists approach the heart indirectly and only from the outside; with the help of technology, they create diagnoses which are then passed on to the heart surgeon if an operation should become necessary. The stuff of life for cardiologists includes electrocardiography, heart ultrasound, spiroergometry, heart CT, transesophageal echocardiography and of course cardiac catheter

examinations and other things. Patients with high blood pressure, arrhythmia, myocardial insufficiency, and vascular disease as well as lung tumors and embolism are safe in their hands, as cardiology is a discipline of internal medicine and specializes in the treatment of the cardiovascular system.

One of my brothers is a cardiologist. Once he transferred a very difficult case to me and was part of the operation, even though the secretary had crossed him off the log – two Dr Natours, that had to be a typo, right? Even though my cardiologist brother works with hearts every day, he had never come close to one like here and now in this space capsule (which is what a high-tech operating room reminds me of). He was especially impressed by how sensitively the heart reacted to the smallest touch, how fine the vessels are when one views them through the magnifying glasses instead of from the outside on a monitor in the cardiac catheter lab. Ever since then, he said, he has no longer passed through the catheter tube quite so swiftly, but rather carefully, tentatively, always remembering the "inner view".

I would like for cardiologists to also get to know the heart from the inside during their training. I am sure that a visit to one single heart would suffice to create a lifelong impression.

When a heart attack is suspected, ultrasound and heart catheter examinations are arranged. If a vessel is narrowed or occluded, it can be repaired during a heart catheter examination using a stent: a metal tube is inserted. If the vessel is already too damaged, the patient needs a bypass and is transferred to the heart surgery department. A heart attack patient who gets to the hospital in time has a good chance to get out again soon and continue their life without any big limitations. Frequently a male patient must thank the presence of mind of his wife as she had not hesitated but called emergency quickly.

Whenever we are in trouble and know that we need help, we wisely seek out a specialist. Various campaigns have enlightened the population in the past few years about all kinds of health risks: defibrillators can be found in many public spaces; one knows that for a long-time bowel cancer does not cause discomfort, and that there is not a second to waste to get medical help in the event of a stroke. The same is true for a heart attack which in the end is nothing but a vessel occlusion in the heart. But a public campaign is different from imagining the worst case in private.

We doctors, too, need other people. Heart surgeons can't achieve anything by themselves but need a team for an operation. When we're in trouble, we always need others – and we should make ourselves aware of that as it is an important part of our self-care, and of our social competence in the instances when others need our help. If you encounter a staggering person somewhere, that does not necessarily mean they are drunk. They could have suffered a stroke. And when they put out a hand and ask for help, they may not want a dollar but for you to call an ambulance.

First Aid
We find it relatively easy to accept help when we pay money for it. In that case we don't owe anyone anything. When we go to the doctor too, we can afford to show our need for help without hesitation – after all, this is a specialist who studied their field and gets paid. On the

other hand, some people place great importance on their autonomy. But people need people, from life's beginning to its end. Without our parents' help, we would not have grown up.

In principle, nothing can be said against the attempt to escape dependency by striving for the utmost autonomy – if we are aware that we are social beings with a social brain. Our brain has grown so big in order for us to get along better in a group. It maneuvers us through millions or even billions of sensory stimuli, checks and roughly sorts them, makes connections, sorts more finely and promptly reach conclusions which guide our behavior. All this occurs from one millisecond to the next, around the clock. Our brain has a heavy workload – and we are not aware of it at all.

If we weren't part of a group, we'd be exposed to all dangers without protection. Humans are social beings and need the contact with others like we need air to breathe; we are not made to be alone.

And yet it is the most horrible thought for many to depend on others. In a crisis or during an illness this is precisely what occurs, sometimes in such an extreme way that we need others to help us eat and go to the toilet. And that can happen to any of us. We can prepare for it without crying wolf. One can think it through. To stipulate one's thoughts about life-extending measures in a living will is to do one's relatives a kindness as they will not have to decide something they are not entitled to decide. This is about taking responsibility for oneself.

4

THE CRASH

Some time ago I travelled to China with a few colleagues to advise health professionals there who were planning for a big heart and vessel center. I could not imagine a replica of our system would work there, because we work from a different normal. That meant we would either have to adjust our approach or train the Chinese colleagues at our own center for a period of time. I was aware of that. Once on the ground I was surprised, despite my doubts, how chaotic this Chinese hospital was – well "chaotic" is my interpretation of it anyway. For example, it was normal in China not to have a waiting area, but people were higgledy-piggledy sitting on the floor. The hospital was functioning nevertheless, like it does in many countries even though they don't follow German standards.

The flight to China, too, had not gone according to German standards. My seat had been double-booked.

The captain himself apologized to me. We liked each other straight away, and he invited me to experience the flight in the so-called jump seat in the cockpit. What a marvelous offer!

With great interest I followed the preparations before take-off. Ah, they had a checklist here in the cockpit, too, just like we did in the operating room. I remembered reading somewhere that the checklists for medical operations had been modelled on those in aviation. The medical lists may sound banal, but in the end, they save lives when we discuss them as a team before an operation.

"We're doing a knee operation", the surgeon says.

Everyone nods.

"It is the right knee", the surgeon adds.

Everyone repeats: "The right knee."

That reduces the probability of operating on the left knee to nearly zero. As a safety measure, the right knee has also been marked. Such measures were established in response to disastrous mistakes. A checklist helps exclude many disastrous errors.

Maybe you are old enough to remember the aviation disaster on Tenerife in 1977. Wikipedia knows it exactly:

On March 27, 1977, two Boeing 747 passenger jets, operating KLM Flight 4805 and Pan Am Flight 1736, collided. (...) Resulting in 583 fatalities, the Tenerife airport disaster is the deadliest in aviation history. (...) The collision occurred when the KLM airliner initiated its take-off run while the Pan Am airliner, shrouded in fog, was still on the runway and about to turn off onto the taxiway. The impact and resulting fire killed everyone on board KLM 4805 and most of the occupants of Pan Am 1736, with only 61 survivors in the front section of the aircraft. The subsequent investigation by Spanish authorities concluded that the primary cause of the accident was the KLM captain's decision to take off in the mistaken belief that a take-off clearance from air traffic control (ATC) had been issued. Dutch investigators placed a greater emphasis on a mutual misunderstanding in radio communications between the KLM crew and ATC. (...)

The disaster had a lasting influence on the industry, highlighting in particular the vital importance of using standardized phraseology in radio communications. Cockpit procedures were also reviewed, contributing to the establishment of crew resource management as a fundamental part of airline pilots' training.[1]

Similar things have occurred in hospitals, too, and today an operation without a checklist is unthinkable. I am convinced that checklists provide a great service during crises. But you have to compile them in advance. A crisis squad which defines its task during a crisis is formed too late. It is better to prepare for all eventualities in advance, as described impressively by Oliver Schneider, a former member of the KSK[2] and a security, risk and crisis management adviser. In his book *Der Wille entscheidet* [The Will Decides], he writes:

"A crisis is an attack on everyday affairs: a new unusual situation for which initially one does not have a plan. That is why one is unsure at the start as to how to behave, which may result in fatal mistakes when desperately trying out solutions and flight options – which in turn leads to deeper and deeper entanglement, constraining oneself and losing room to maneuver. There is no fallback experience for this emergency."

All types of crises follow a certain sequence. There may be many people involved or a few, a whole country may be implicated or a family, a relationship, matters of health or finance. The future is in danger. One does not know how life will go on. What was valid only yesterday is uncertain today.

What is to be done? How does one behave correctly? Is one able to influence the course of things at all? A checklist can support us in our role as crisis navigators. We can create our own list for emergencies. That is enormously important, because once in trouble we may not be able to think clearly anymore. Terrible things may occur when we're in panic mode, things we would never have done with a clear mind. Most people remember one situation or another in which they did or said things they later regretted.

"It was as if I'd lost my mind." – "I was beside myself." A crime of passion, as they say in detective stories.

We are indeed "beside ourselves" in an emergency situation. But if we define a checklist for ourselves, we are unlikely to stay like that for long. Dealing with crises can be practiced by not getting too cozy in one's comfort zone, and instead reminding oneself every now and then that there is no right to one's normal and that crises are part of life. They rarely occur suddenly, most of them have a prehistory. It is part of crisis management to try and develop a seismographic perception of such prehistory as early as possible. On the other hand, spending a lot of time on defense mechanisms may negatively influence the outcome.

Once the crisis breaks out, chaos reigns at first and seems for some time be the new normal – yet it is merely a bridge. Our first steps during this time will determine our direction, our plan to master the crisis. A person who is prepared will find this easier to do. But they are not alone, and a team is only as good as its weakest member.

That is why everyone involved will have to adjust to the changed situation – and that, as we have recently experienced all over the world, may take time.

The checklist

With the COVID-19 crisis, we realized how much chaos is unleashed when there are no checklists to ensure a clear plan of action. Virologists and other health professionals as well as veterinarians and various other specialists had warned time and time again that we are headed for a pandemic. But their voices were not heard. Now, after the COVID-19 experience, there is already some talk about how we should expect the next pandemic. Some people are working on the improvement of procedures so that next time things go more smoothly. It seems to be the case again and again that the first or maybe also the second knock on the door is not heard: the door must be broken down, which sometimes means that the whole house collapses.

And when we are affected by an illness ourselves? The earth seems to open up, especially when an examination brings an accidental diagnosis which is terrible. The ground beneath our feet shakes, everything caves in. The quicker we get back onto solid ground, the better. In such a case, a checklist really has the role of life insurance. I mean that literally: we make sure that we are still alive. We fall into a hole, yes, but we look for a rope ladder, for people who can help us. It may take a fair bit of time, but to have looked ahead gives us a good feeling. Like in an operating room, where checklists are called briefings. During a briefing, we go through standard procedures as well as various scenarios, so that we are all at the same level of knowledge: what have we planned, what do we specifically need to look out for, what happens if plan A does not work and plan B does not work either and so on.

Have we discussed how to position the patient?
Have we discussed the operating time?
Is the correct operating table available?
Are all apparatuses and instruments ready to go?
Do we have the correct implants and prostheses?
Have specific safety measures been discussed?
Is blood coagulation good?
Which temperature will we go for?
Will we shut down the heart?
If so, will we also shut down blood circulation?
And if so, how will we provide blood for the brain?
How exactly will we connect the patient to the heart-lung machine?
Is a postoperative bed available in the ICU?

We could, no, should be the first people to ask these questions, because if no bed is available in ICU we can't operate. After the operation the patient will have to be looked after in intensive care. Many people forgot during the COVID-19 crisis that ICU beds are not only needed for COVID-19 patients, but also for everyday proceedings at hospitals: beds for victims of accidents, for people just out of the operating room, for emergencies of all kinds.

What does your checklist look like? What would you want for your own heart? Well, have you ever even been in contact with it?

Heart Talk

Maybe you would like to place a hand on your chest. Do you feel your heartbeat? Stay awhile with your heart and realize that you are the specialist for your heart. Maybe your heart will not yet talk to you the first time. After all, it has been waiting for a long time for you to make contact. How wonderful that you are initiating it, instead of waiting for a cry for help from your heart, a first warning knock. By establishing contact with your heart, you are also establishing contact with yourself. You collect yourself; you explore what's inside you. More and more people practice mindfulness exercises like yoga and other relaxation techniques to create for themselves an island in these wild, hectic times. An island of relaxation to which you can return again and again. Those who practice this for a long time will stand securely and safely in life and will not be so readily knocked over, not even by a crisis.

To start yoga when the crisis has already arrived isn't bad, but it would be better to have started already. Thus, one dot point on your checklist could be to mention things you are doing today to be able to confront unforeseen events which may unsettle your life tomorrow or the day after.

	1	2	3	4	5	6	7
In most ways my life is close to my ideal.	○	○	○	○	○	○	○
The conditions of my life are excellent.	○	○	○	○	○	○	○
I am satisfied with my life.	○	○	○	○	○	○	○
So far, I have gotten the important things I want in life.	○	○	○	○	○	○	○
If I could live my life over, I would change almost nothing.	○	○	○	○	○	○	○

- 7 - Strongly agree
- 6 - Agree
- 5 - Slightly agree
- 4 - Neither agree nor disagree
- 3 - Slightly disagree
- 2 - Disagree
- 1 - Strongly disagree

In medicine worldwide, the SF-36 questionnaire is used to determine people's quality of life:[3]

The five questions of the *Satisfaction with Life Scale Test* of American psychologists Diener, Emmons, Larsen and Griffin may provide a first step towards a conversation with yourself. It is a test used frequently around the globe to determine how satisfied you are with life, enabling you to find out quickly and straightforwardly where you stand regarding the question "How am I?"

You can find this questionnaire on the website of one of its original creators, Ed Diener. On the same page, you can find translations of the test into over thirty languages as well as a section which explains the scoring for the test.[4]

[1]   https://en.wikipedia.org/wiki/ Tenerife_airport_disaster

[2] Kommando Spezialkräfte, the special forces command of the Bundeswehr, the German army.

[3]   https://heartbeat-med.com/resources/short-form-36-sf-36

[4]   http://labs.psychology.illinois.edu/~ediener/ SWLS.html

5

A CLEAR HEAD
IN THE CRISIS

How capable are you of handling an emergency? Can you
work towards a goal outside of the normal circumstances
you are used to? Even though the onset of an illness may
initially paralyze you, working towards a goal is
necessary in the long run, because if we continue to feel
powerless and unable to act, we will feel stressed
permanently – and that is not good.

Let us board a plane again. Before take-off, the
passengers receive instructions for an emergency. No
one believes it will happen, except maybe the pale young
man with cold sweat on his forehead in row twelve –
and yet everyone nods when they are told where the life
jackets are and how they are inflated. Assuming there
would be an emergency… those who paid attention
would be at an advantage – and still in grave danger, as

those who did not pay attention would panic and mess everything up. After all they have no idea what to do. They may block the exits, thrash about wildly, freeze or collapse.

In a hospital, we have more time than during a plane crash. Through a series of conversations, we can reach even those patients who weren't paying attention at the start and did not want to deal with the fact that they'd have to put on a life jacket.

"But I've always been in good health!"

Yes. Until now. But your health of the past does not mean it will remain with you forever and a day. The conversations at the start of an illness are enormously important for patients not to crash but instead keep a clear head in the crisis, so they know where the life jacket is, how to inflate it and where the exits are located. In most cases patients discuss this with their families. Fellow patients may inspire them, too, fellow sufferers from whom one can learn as they may provide a different view of things. But nothing can replace a conversation with a trusted doctor. I believe that many health professionals are not even aware of the huge influence they exercise on the course of the crisis through their behavior and their care. What may at first glance constitute a considerable effort, will save much time and money in the long run – because patients who feel well looked after reacting to the treatment differently: when they say yes to the medical measures, no energy is wasted. Stress drains us of energy.

Stress Makes You Sick

"I am stressed", you hear everywhere. A stress reaction

signifies the body's adjustment to exceptional challenges to allow us to master dangerous situations. In the short run, that's a great thing. In the long run, we have to avoid it – something that has become increasingly difficult as on the whole we are a stressed society, even though stress is no longer *en vogue* and people usually emphasize that they are completely relaxed. Stress is only for people who have lost control over their lives, right? And so, we feel stressed because it stresses us that the others might notice that we're stressed.

Stress does not only mean that one is overworked and likes to do, or should do, or has to do, too many things at once. Stress is another word for certain physical processes, and it is those processes which cause us to feel stressed. The triggers for stress are as diverse as life: moving house, a pandemic, an unpleasant phone call, a divorce, a colleague, an illness, vague fears. If all goes well, the cortisol level that rose during a stress attack drops again little by little. If the stress level remains high, it means danger for the person as the high cortisol level leads to further physical reactions which are not conducive to one's health in the long run. In a crisis, the stress level remains very high over a longer period of time and thus exacerbates the crisis as continuing stress is detrimental for most of our organs and changes our hormone and nervous systems. If there are no phases of recovery, one may even die early.

Important indicators of the onset of stress are loss of control and hopelessness: when people have the feeling they can no longer control and plan their lives and when they believe that this is not going to change in the near future. Fears also kick in, even fear of death. Stress can increase anxiety as the glucocorticoid receptors for the stress hormone cortisol convey a heightened sense of fear. We feel fear in our bodies, regardless of the reasons for it being real or irrational. Our heartbeat and breathing accelerate, our perspiratory glands increase production, our mouth becomes dry, our hands shake and most importantly – our ability to think clearly is blocked. Instead of being able to make constructive decisions, we are paralyzed by a vague sensation or lapse into a state of shock. Even those who have both feet on the ground, as they say, do not know how they would react in exceptional circumstances. That is why specialists (for example, members of the special forces or extreme athletes or surgeons) frequently practice situations out of the ordinary to integrate them into their everyday work and to minimize the danger of making mistakes due to stress. When stressed we are not masters of ourselves. We know this from the animal kingdom, too: in an emergency an animal will flee, lapse into a state of shock or attack. All of us can remember situations from their life in which they reacted in one of these three ways, afterwards maybe asking themselves: "How could I?"

It is of course not a nice task to imagine oneself in a crisis or seriously ill. But the knowledge that we may become paralyzed in an emergency may motivate us to think about it all in advance – simply because as human beings we must accept that stress may block our ability to act and to assess a situation accurately. In a stressful situation, our perception of the environment may change. The brain switches to its emergency mode when it notices danger, and stress signals danger. The hormones adrenaline and noradrenaline are released. Additional air is sucked into our lungs to provide the blood with sufficient oxygen and pump it more quickly to the muscles of our upper arms and thighs rather than our brain, which facilitates our reaction of either fleeing or attacking; this gives us more strength. At the same time, bodily functions which aren't of any use when we're in danger are reduced or switched off completely. Unfortunately, this also diminishes our complex thinking.

These physical processes were lifesaving for our ancestors: "Let's get out of here!" or "Hit it!" For us, however, they are no longer constructive. On the other hand, as these processes occur unconsciously, they are not controllable. Yet if we know that they are automated, we can react accordingly. For what good is it to us if, after receiving bad news, we remain in a physical state as if we were fleeing, or frozen with shock and unable to act for days.

If we make ourselves aware of the strength required by a permanent stress mode, we understand the importance of lowering the stress level during a crisis. For surgical interventions, good psychological preparation for the planned operation can help reduce postoperative complications. Studies about surgical patients reveal that those who report increased stress levels on day three after the operation will suffer longer stays in hospital, a higher complication rate and wound healing disorders after interventions such as gall bladder or bypass operations. It was further observed that the time for wound healing increases up to four times for frightened and depressive patients, compared to those who are better able to come to terms with the psychological strain of stress.

A patient in need of lots of care, by the way, also puts

stress on the staff. Less and less staff for more and more patients – a dilemma which rather often plays out at the expense of those who once joined the profession highly motivated and ready to help, who are now being used: it is them, after all, who are on the frontline and have to say no. How is this meant to work, how can one leave work feeling good, knowing one should have stayed in the ward for at least another two hours to get everything done that needed doing, including holding a patient's hand. But one had already extended one's shift by one hour... Here we clearly see how the desire to save time and money leads into a dangerous dead-end street; as a society, we should be aware of this. After all, one of our most pressing questions is: how do we want to shape the medicine of the future?

COVID-19 turned many dormant embers which had been smoldering for a long time into large-scale fires. Nursing staff is becoming scarcer and scarcer because people have worked at their limit for too long and eventually can't do it anymore – and their work is not even paid adequately. Less staff means less beds, less beds means less operations, and less operations means sicker people and...dead ones.

The point in time when someone's warning light starts to flash is different from person to person. That is exactly what we want to determine for each patient at our clinic in Maastricht, to become able to meet our patients where they are at. Every person's resilience is different and depends not only on their physical constitution but many other additional factors: how we feel on a particular day, how we slept, our hormone levels, the state of our relationship, the weather and so on. Nevertheless, one can find out in a conversation how robust and resilient a patient is. Our aim is to stress them as little as possible, as stress is counterproductive for the course of their illness. Of course, we cannot keep their stay in the hospital entirely stress-free, but we determine what we can and cannot expect of them. It is surprising which degrading situations are forced upon patients in everyday medicine – and hardly anyone seems to notice. In our clinic we encourage patients to consider alternative paths. Ideally, they would have worked on those before when they compiled their individual checklist. An important point here is to remind patients – and they should be doing this of their own accord – of difficult situations they have mastered well in the past. They should concentrate on those successes. Our problem-solving ability and our confidence can soothe our immune system.

A sentence like "I'm sure this is not the first difficult situation in your life" can prompt a patient to think about it and give them strength. A short sentence which can have lasting implications.

The relatives, too, should be aware of how important it is to protect patients from stress. Surely, they'll say: "Now you see that you get better", but it is not so rare for them to approach the sick bed with questions that will strain the patients even though they don't want to let on about it. That occurs most often with the wives of a generation which was used to the husbands making all decisions and is now completely overwhelmed, therefore bringing many everyday issues into the hospital: "The heating does not work, what should I do about the insurance, the lawn mower is broken." And he is in his sick bed, despairing because he is no longer of any use – and even more so as it is made so abundantly clear to them, even though it happens with the best intentions: *I need you*. Ideally families bubble-wrap the patients in a stress-free space and keep anything alarming away from them.

There are also people who will not get into situations where they are stressed by their relatives as they have little contact with their families. Yet one can feel lonely with lots of contact, too, even lonelier, for example, if one is afraid of an operation but is unable to say so, pretending to be strong but feeling like crying. No one understands. The world is on its head. That, too, is a deep experience of loneliness.

Data from millions of people show that those who feel lonely are 30 to 50 percent more likely to die, which probably makes their mortality risk bigger than that of smokers, alcoholics, or severely obese people, as Prof Bettina M Pause explains in her book *Alles Geruchssache* [It's All a Matter of Smell]. Furthermore, loneliness is one of the most important causes for a plethora of mental disorders, among them anxiety disorders, depression, dementia or schizophrenia. Social isolation and loneliness lead humans to mental disorders and early death so effectively and immediately like hardly any other issues. Loneliness is pure stress. Stress research mentions the permanent feeling of having no control over important aspects of one's life, especially regarding the all-important relationships with others, who can be happy with us and be by our side when we suffer. What we need most during a crisis is closeness to others, especially if we are seriously ill. And it is wonderful when those who are with us can wrap us in cotton wool for a while until we are able to power up the lawn mower again.

The Height of the Fall

We have talked about how each person deals differently with a crisis, a serious misfortune, or a severe illness. The height of the fall plays an important role here. If someone crashes down from a beautiful plenteous life and so far, has had little experience with downfalls and failures, they hit the ground harder – they fall from the roof terrace. Someone else does not live that high up, just on the third floor; they have not quite that far to fall. Those living on the first floor may just shrug and think: well, I didn't need this right now on top of everything else.

When in contact with someone who is affected, however, we cannot just say: "pull yourself together… you've had such a nice life up on your roof terrace, sun from morning to evening… others live in the basement and never had that pleasure". The patients from the roof terrace have the problem that they don't know their way around down there on the ground – but maybe they have a crisis navigator and are prepared for this event by means of a checklist for the worst-case scenario. The key question is: what do we expect from ourselves when trying to master this challenge?

Someone who is used to living on the sunny side of life will sometimes have great difficulty to admit to themselves and others that they are now in the shadow. It is helpful in this regard to question one's expectations critically. Often this will lead to the insight that one is not quite so fully in control of life as one thought. That can be painful but also liberating; we realize there are certain things which are out of our hands. Other matters, however, *are* in our hands – namely how we deal with changes and if we insist on the roof terrace or can imagine living comfortably on the first floor. With a garden, of course! In a pinch a fantasy garden will do, as we can make it as lush as we want.

When doctors enlighten their patients about how the illness or operation will change their lives, they often only mention losses – like a banker who advises his clients after the crash to stake their future no longer on the Ferrari but the bicycle. That may well be important as we don't want to sugarcoat the facts – but we should not be fixated on the deficit but help patients develop new perspectives as much as possible. We will not only lose but also gain – and how we embrace and integrate that will decide how our life will continue.

In times of change, we concentrate generally on the things we will lose. We have forgotten that nothing in life is forever. A crisis can teach us to accept change as a part of life. Regarding illnesses, this also means that we do not only regard them as a sort of transitional stage in the aging process (after all, don't old and sick go together?), but focus on our abilities. Some of them we will only discover over time, and only if we are open to recognizing them. You cannot reverse a severe illness. You cannot reverse bankruptcy. But how we shape our life afterwards is in our own hands. However, that requires us to accept change rather than wanting to go back to the roof terrace at all costs.

If we recount our life when we're advanced in years, we may be astonished to see how often we have changed our residence. From the roof terrace into the basement, into a bungalow and finally into a private residence…then later into a place on the second floor, which isn't a problem as we have experience with various domiciles. Variety makes life interesting. In retrospect, crises are the most exciting episodes – if we have mastered them well, that is. We learn from people who have taken a deep fall: how did they pick themselves up? They can be our role model. Hey, there is a beautiful life away from the roof terrace... and maybe the first-floor apartment with a shared garden won't be the right home anymore after a while...let's move to a houseboat!

When we defend our normality against the change of life, we utilize only very few of our opportunities. There are so many ways to shape our life! I learned this from patients who succeeded in creating a new abundance from deficit. Like gardener Kurt Peipe, who received his diagnosis of bowel cancer when he was sixty-five and set off – with an ostomy – on foot from the German/ Danish border to Assisi in Italy. He told no one how seriously ill he was; he did not want compassion. He marched for thirty or forty kilometers each day, slept in a tent which he was sometimes allowed to pitch in the garden of someone who would also feed him. At first, he declined, but then realized that by doing so he was rejecting friendliness and generosity – and that it does both sides good when offerings are accepted. The father of three learned a lot about life and people. His illness opened a new horizon for him. When he reached his destination, Assisi, he had become a new person. And this new person he had gained through his hike was so precious to him that he said: "If I had the choice to have no cancer and live like before, or to have cancer but also everything I was allowed to experience in the last few months – then I would take the new Kurt." Shortly before his death he wrote a very readable book (now unfortunately out of print) about his hike: *Dem Leben auf den Fersen* [On the Heels of Life].[1]

People who survive a crisis or illness also often say that

in retrospect they are thankful for this time as otherwise they would never have arrived where the crisis or illness led them. Such a path may be painful while you're on it. I know patients who have not only lost a heart valve but also their life partner who could not deal with the situation. But maybe they found new love or got to know themselves anew and realized they cope better by themselves. In any case... people for whom the glass is half full will always find a narrative where everything worked out well in the end. Life is easier for them, similar to those who have the ability to call on resources from the past. Sometimes people learn to do this only during an illness. They recognize how precious life is and how nonsensical it is to spoil it with so many silly trifles. A severe illness may help some of us find our way in life, leading to a better future. Today we sow the seeds that will help us deal with crises tomorrow and the day after, so that at such time we can remember that today – which by then will have become yesterday – we mastered the challenge and have grown because of it.

Sure, this is the ideal scenario. There are many stumbling stones on the way to mastering a crisis. But it is good to realize that despite all the terrible things we can't control, our attitude towards the situation is up to us alone. And that is at least half the rent for the roof terrace!

[1] https://www.sueddeutsche.de/panorama/kurt-peipe-eine-geschichte-die-das-leben-schrieb-1.700984   (in German).

6

THE IMPACT

The use of ever more imaging technologies in medicine has led to large numbers of incidental findings. During an ultrasound of the upper abdomen a liver cyst is diagnosed; an x-ray of the spine brings to light a tumor. The discovery of a very dangerous time bomb, namely the dilation of a blood vessel, is one such accidental finding. In the past such an aneurysm was mostly identified too late, while today we can see it during an ultrasound or x-ray. The abdominal aorta is affected most frequently, but mammary and cerebral arteries can be concerned too. An operation becomes the treatment of choice once the aneurysm reaches a certain size, as a tear would result in life-threatening bleedings. Patients won't know the danger they are in because aneurysms often do not cause any discomfort; if on the other hand they feel discomfort (for example a cough, indigestion, a headache) it can't be assigned to its cause.

If the blood vessel tears, the pain is excruciating, often likened to an elephant sitting on someone's chest. Circulatory collapse and coma may follow.

Medicine can prevent such a rude awakening by using a stent during a heart catheter examination or a bypass operation. If an aneurysm is diagnosed in time and if the patients regularly come to follow-up examinations, they have good chances given their blood pressure is normal (which can also be achieved by medication). If an aneurysm tears, the chances are fifty-fifty.

Usually aneurysms grow slowly, one to two millimeters a year, but growth spurts may occur and then the day has come when a patient will be transferred to the vessel or heart surgery ward. The risk of the vessel wall tearing increases as soon as an aortic aneurysm reaches a diameter of five and a half centimeters in the chest. The life-saving operation is difficult because the vessel may also tear during the intervention. With an aneurysm in the brain, the risk is even higher, and irreversible brain damage may occur.

I am very experienced in aortic surgery and have been able to help many people. Such operations are much more challenging compared, for example, to a bypass procedure or changing a heart valve – even though I wouldn't call these routine procedures either. From the patient's point of view no intervention is ever routine.

With many illnesses, patients suffer discomfort and sometimes such strong pain that they are longing for the operation. With aneurysms, however, they often feel fit and have come to see the doctor about a different matter – and then within minutes change from a healthy person to someone gravely ill or even moribund when they are told: "We have to operate as soon as possible, otherwise..." In no time at all their normal life ceases to exist – everything changes and nothing is valid anymore. The vacation, the relocation, the weekend, the children's graduation... everything is different.

"Can we postpone this?", the patients sometimes ask because the urgency is not clear to them. They simply can't imagine this when they feel so well.

If the answer is "I'd rather not", I have usually been informed already, or else a colleague when I'm not on duty. In some cases, we operate on the same day or the next morning, hardly leaving any time to talk to the relatives. You can compare it to an accident which also hits you unexpectedly. Someone got into their car fit as a fiddle, and two hours later is rushed to hospital with flashing ambulance lights: head-on collision, resuscitation area, emergency operation.

If the patient is conscious, a conversation with the doctor is immensely important in order to take away fear, paint a realistic picture of the situation, and above all get to know each other. This is the surgeon who will operate on me in the morning. And the other way around: this is the person whose heart I will hold in my hands tomorrow. This knowledge continues to resonate even when one then discusses general matters – details of the operation, possible complications, an assessment of the risk and the question what would happen if the operation was not done.

Tomorrow, you will cut me open and will look deep inside like no one else can, not even me.

Are you a good surgeon?

Will you not have one drink too many today, go to bed early to be fit in the morning?

How often have you done this already?
How many patients have died under your hands?
Can I trust you?

All these questions cross my mind, too. Yes, I am a good surgeon, and I absolutely won't drink too much, I will go to bed early and try to be in top shape tomorrow. It will be an adventure for me as well: even after thousands of operations this one procedure tomorrow is special. It is potentially the biggest crisis in my patient's life, and once I hold the scalpel in my hand tomorrow, I will be a part of this crisis. We are in the same boat.

I feel it when patients give me their Yes. That is always a special moment. It is not talked about, yet is palpable. I really regret it when there is only little time before an operation, when acute danger urges us to act quickly. In such cases the time to deal with things, for which others have days and weeks, is reduced to mere hours. Some patients prefer that, albeit only in retrospect – when they have spoken to fellow sufferers in their ward who had prepared weeks or months for the intervention. From them they hear that is not an untroubled time as the operation's sword of Damocles is hanging over you. On the other hand, this time can be used, for example to compile a checklist and to steady oneself with relaxation techniques, yoga, meditation and so on. Dancing is recommended, too, music, walks, Tai chi, Qigong… the possibilities have become so numerous that there is something for everyone.

When a patient asks me: "How will I feel after the intervention?", I often have to say, regrettably: "Worse than now."

That is the crazy thing. The patient is well, has no discomfort. The danger to their life was discovered by accident. That reminds one a little of cancer therapy when patients often do not know that there is a malignant tumor growing inside them. They feel no discomfort, believe they are healthy and look well. Only once medicine rolls out its heavy artillery – that is, during treatment when hopefully their healing has been set in motion – they feel bad, and it shows.

"Doctor, do I understand this correctly – I feel completely healthy, but I am gravely ill, and if I'm not operated on I may be dead tomorrow… even though I'm well. And if I undergo the operation, I will feel worse than now afterwards."

"Yes."

"And if not?"

I'm silent.

"How many percent worse?", the fifty-five-year-old patient asks.

"Ten", I estimate.

He thinks about it. "Ten?"

I nod.

"Well, that's not so bad then."

And he has started to negotiate with his illness. He is ready to accept his fate. It does not always happen this quickly, and a Yes may be withdrawn. Five minutes later, a patient may have doubts. It goes back and forth, up and down – that is the sign of a crisis.

The Five Phases of Coming to Terms with an Illness

These five phases can be traced back to an internationally known death researcher, Elisabeth Kübler-Ross. That may sound strange for a moment, but her findings can be transferred to every crisis, in particular to dealing with an illness. Many people suffer from extreme mood swings during such a time. They no longer know themselves. Like in a roller-coaster ride they go up and down, up and down. It relieves them to find out that this is normal when one's normal life ceases to exist.

The five phases are not a timetable out of the crises; there is no well-timed succession but rather some chaotic traffic. However, there are five main roads on which we travel through our crises. We cross other roads, leave paths, go back, and start again. If you make yourself aware of these five phases, you will gain and retain orientation much more easily. You can trust the fact that you are already actively engaged with the crisis on the inside, even though outwardly it does not appear like that.

The first phase: shock

After getting the diagnosis, we are often unable to grasp what we heard. We believe and hope there's a mistake – wrong results from the lab maybe? We have always led a healthy life after all. "Why me?" Maybe we feel no pain whatsoever and thus can't connect the results of the examination with ourselves. People in this first phase compare it to having fallen into a big hole, from the bottom of which they are facing a huge climb, and the ground beneath their feet is shaking. Nothing is valid anymore.

The second phase: suppression

What has crashed into our lives is too powerful for us.

We cannot digest it. We fight against it, do not want to accept it, maybe we deny it. This phase, which contains moments of reluctant understanding of the new reality, somehow helps us. The news is too gigantic for us to grasp it all at once. Through the seesaw of our emotions, we digest it in smaller pieces which we can absorb more easily.

The third phase: wild emotions

We are furious, annoyed, scornful, despondent, sad – all at once. Tossed around by our emotions, we may become unfair towards others. We are strangers to ourselves, lost in the jungle of extreme emotions and possibly impatient, unreasonable – at times making it hard for those who want to help us, which we later regret.

Relatives and friends, too, live through this phase. They are also affected, after all, even though they are not patients themselves. In some way, they must deal with a double crisis.

If, as relatives, we understand that the not-so-nice reactions in the process of coping with a crisis stem not so much from the patient but rather the illness, we can deal with them more easily ourselves. Patience is of the essence here – patience with oneself and with others. The sick person's occasional rude manners should not be taken personally.

Some people are battered by existential despair, while others withdraw during this phase, hardly talking anymore, gliding into a depression. Because what are they worth now, as a sick person? Self-doubts eat away at them. Within the circle of family and friends, this is a difficult situation which requires a lot of understanding, tactfulness, and yes, love. Should the relatives retreat aggrieved, it will become a lot worse for everyone.

Make yourself aware: this is only a phase, even though you cannot imagine at the moment that you will ever emerge from it.

Fourth phase: action and negotiation

Now we become active again. We tackle the illness. We try to set in motion everything that is possible to master the challenges, we make sure to obtain information, talk to others, explore alternative paths. Maybe we undertake a pilgrimage, talk to God, look for signs that all will turn out well. We want to make a deal with fate: "If I get better, I promise that I…"

Fifth phase: acceptance

Gradually we manage to process the illness emotionally. By and by we find paths to a new normality, at least if things are going well. Sometimes that does not work as the acceptance of an illness does not appear automatically; it depends on different factors. Often patients remain trapped in the first four phases, unable to find an exit. In such cases, a hint can sometimes help which could provide motivation for the patient to take the next step and accept the new normal.

That would be healthier, in any case, not only for the patient but also for their family and friends. I remember a sixty-year-old patient who after a heart attack and resuscitation turned into a gruff, abrasive, bad-tempered person who made his family and especially his wife suffer badly. Even though he had good chances of recovery if he accepted the offers for rehabilitation, he rejected everything. He did not want to have had a heart attack, did not want anything to do with all this nonsense, end of story. Never in a million years would he turn into a clown in a cardiac rehab group or talk to a psychologist – why, he wasn't crazy. In any case he did not know why his wife and two daughters were continuously interfering. His wife wished with all her heart for him to accept his illness, as only in that way they would be able to begin again together. In the end the woman suffered so badly from the stubborn behavior of her husband that her own heart became ill. Even that did not bring her husband to concede. Her daughters told me in an email that tragically their mother then suffered a serious heart attack and died at the clinic. My former patient, who could not manage his life without his wife, had to be moved to a nursing home.

How long it takes to live through the aforementioned five phases is different for every person, for every patient. It also depends on the severity of the illness, the occurrence of setbacks and so on. For many patients it is a relief if they no longer feel that they are simply at the mercy of their chaotic emotions but can distinguish a structure. Chaos is part of crisis management, part of a good path to recovery – even though it may not feel like that at the moment.

We cannot turn back the clock on an illness, but we can learn to live with it and create a new normal.

The Cooled-down Patient

Luca, one of my patients, had to adjust very early to a new normal which had been curtailed by illness. This new normal had now become fragile again. I had operated on this Italian man, now aged thirty-six, eight years earlier when he had been studying in Germany.

As a Marfan patient he needed a second operation: it occurs rather frequently with this inherited disease that the aorta needs to be replaced piece by piece.

Marfan patients suffer from a weakness of the connective tissue. As connective tissue can be found everywhere in our body, many organs and body structures are affected – very often it is the heart and the vessels, and particularly the main artery, the aorta. The degree of danger is assessed according to where it tears. If the tear is in the carotid arteries, a stroke or brain death can result. If it tears near the heart, affecting the coronary artery, a severe heart attack can occur. The tear causes the aortic valve to lose its attachment to the aortic wall and begin to leak. This causes massive problems for the heart as it is no longer able to properly pump away the blood. It can also happen that so much blood flows into the heart sac that the heart drowns in its own blood, unable to pump. That is a death sentence.

When I first met Luca, the twenty-eight-year-old's aorta had torn even though he was under a tight monitoring regime and had his aorta checked out every few months. At least he was able to interpret the excruciating pain. With my team I managed to save his life for the time being. He owes the fact that his life became so beautiful again afterwards not only to himself but to many people who supported him at our clinic, during rehab and in his circle of friends.

Unfortunately, trouble wasn't over for Luca after this big eight-hour operation. The rest of his aorta continued to become affected and now threatened to explode, quite literally. After an operation, adhesions usually form in the tissue. Normally the aorta is positioned under the sternum, but if it has been operated on, the adhesions practically attach it to the sternum. If I were to saw my patient's sternum open, I would saw directly into the aorta; that would be a disaster. You can stem bleeding by putting a finger into the hole. But sometimes one finger is not sufficient, it needs to be two or three – but there is not enough space for them, and the hole is expanding so the patient is losing more and more blood. If the heart becomes emptier and emptier, it can no longer pump properly. This is one of the instances one would rather only think through in theory. But they occur, and then one has to act very quickly – or else one has worked on one's checklist meticulously so risks like this are excluded in the first place.

But we have a checklist which quickly reveals such risks, so we can switch to Plan B: to connect the patient immediately to the heart-lung machine, using the groin vessels which are often used to access the body, for example in a heart catheter examination.

Today we can even insert heart valves through the groin; this relatively new procedure is called TAVI, *Transcatheter Aortic Valve Implantation.*

While our anesthetist is sending Luca into the land of dreams, I will briefly tell you something about heart valves. They are among the most mechanically strained parts of our body. They open and close with every heartbeat and control the bloodstream through our heart like mechanical valves, one hundred thousand times a day. The aortic valve is especially strained in this process. At the point of transition from the left ventricle into the aorta, it controls the flow of the blood rich in oxygen from the heart into the body. If the valve is calcified or hardened (which may occur with increasing age or for other reasons), the heart muscle has to pump more strongly, which decreases a patient's performance: they complain about shortness of breath when they exercise, about heart pain and dizziness. In some cases, the valve will have to be replaced, which was for many decades done by opening the sternum while the heart was shut down. The heart-lung machine took over the job. TAVI has for some time now provided us with a gentler possibility for inoperable high-risk patients and the elderly. We don't even require general anesthetic as the procedure takes place under local anesthesia. A new heart valve in the morning, back at home in the evening.

My patient Luca could only dream about something like that. He was facing a much more serious operation than "merely" the implantation of a new valve.

Wednesday, 8.50am

Luca has been wired up and is sleeping on the operating table. Once more I make sure that everyone in the team is ready, has done the last check, has studied my drawings on the whiteboard (which depict how things look inside the patient now and how they are meant to look after the operation). Now we transform Luca's body as well as our own and the environment of the operating table into a sterile area. While my assistant and I wash, our patient is washed and covered. The tubes of the heart-lung machine are fixed to the drapes.

Beeps sound in the operating room. Beep, beep, beep…this sound will be with us for the coming hours. It is a good sound, signaling to us that all is well. Should it change dramatically, we will be on the alert. Beep, beep, beep…about fifty times every minute. The heart is beating more slowly than usually because of the anesthetic.

"May we begin?", I ask the anesthetist.

"Yes, we can begin."

We apply a five-centimeter cut in the groin, exposing the vessels. The patient's blood has been heavily thinned with heparin to avoid clotting. We connect the cannulas for the vessels to the tubes of the heart-lung machine. The cardiac technician (also called perfusionist) announces: "Machine connected, no problems, full flow!"

The machine has taken over now. The heart is still working, but has no duties to perform. We begin to cool the patient down. As we expect adhesions and other difficulties in the thorax, we need to go down to 22°C (71.6°F). The scar above Luca's sternum is cut out, the old steel wires are removed. I open the sternum with a surgical saw, because in its middle the aorta is attached to the bone. The perfusionist stops the heart-lung machine at 28°C (82.4°F), which takes the pressure off the aorta so we can open the sternum. This happens incredibly fast as the patient has no blood pressure. The aorta is open and is quickly detached from the bone. Blood suction keeps our field of vision clear. We suture the defect in the aorta which we had to cause as it was attached to the bone – that is why it was so important to quickly attach the patient to the heart-lung machine, which is our safety net.

The actual operation is still ahead of Luca and us. We restart the heart-lung machine and cool the patient until we reach our goal of 22°C. Three tense minutes. Beep, beep, beep. We take a deep breath...everything's okay again. Fantastic team, I think. Later I will say it. But now we concentrate on the next steps. The carotid arteries and the aortic arch are exposed, including the section at the start of the aorta where I operated eight years ago. We see the old prosthesis. Looks good. Today we will replace

Luca's aortic arch. We will also prepare everything for the third operation – his descending aorta will additionally have to be replaced down to his abdomen within the next few years. At the end of his life, hopefully a long one, nearly his whole aorta will have let him down section by section and will have been replaced.

When the temperature has reached 22°C, we shut down Luca's circulation. Three small tubes provide blood through the carotid arteries, supplying the brain with blood while the rest of his body remains without blood.

Now we look into the aorta. The result of the SC scan is confirmed: the aorta is torn, and Luca's tissue is very weak due to his Marfan.

We cut out the aortic arch and will replace it with a combined prosthesis, a dacron part with a stent. The stent is inserted into the descending aorta and released there. It will remain in the aorta, supporting the tissue in this area and at the same time serving as a connector for the next step. As the stent reminds one of an elephant's trunk, this operation method is called *Frozen Elephant Trunk Technique*.

We sew the prosthesis to the surrounding aorta wall. After finishing this connection, called anastomosis, a cannula is fixed to the dacron arm of the prosthesis, and the heart-lung machine starts again to support the body. The temperature of the blood is slowly increased towards 36.5°C (97.7°F).

The next step is to connect the dacron part with the old prosthesis. Now the heart is also connected, vented thoroughly, and allowed to participate again. It shivers with cold and fibrillates. At about 26°C (78.8°F) it can be defibrillated. A pacemaker provides a steady rhythm, and there it is again: beep, beep, beep.

The connection of the carotid arteries to the arch prosthesis constitutes the next challenge. No air must get to the brain! Luca is now warm again; heart and lungs are working well. We start to bring the patient back by reducing the input of the heart-lung machine. The blood thinning is cancelled by a counteragent, protamine. Thorough hemostasis must be conducted. Finally, the cannulas are extracted from the groin vessels and the wound is closed. The anesthetist is very happy as the heart echocardiograph shows the heart is functioning well. The OR nurses have checked the materials and announce: all fine, all stable, all accounted for.

We can close the thorax. The sternum is held together by steel wires, the wound sutured in layers. I step out of the sterile area, take off my gloves and go to the telephone to call Luca's family. After that I will compose a different operation report than the one you just read, one that is peppered with jargon like this:

st n asc replacement 8y ago, now reop FET with prep before TAA.

HLM fem – fem with asc adhesion w sternum.

22° sternum open with aorta at 28°, HLM stop, hole sutured, and HLM on again, cool further

arrest, aorta open, inspection: asc arch, photos, FET, anastomosis, re-canule, HLM start and warm up, connect heart. At 26° defi> SR bradykard, PM, connect to neck vessels.

reperfusion, HLM stop, hemostasis, 3 drainages, 2 pacemakers, wires, thorax closed.

TEE: good heart function biventricular.

CAVE: secondary hemorrhage, high blood pressure.

Family called.

7

PREOPERATIVE CONVERSATION

As mentioned already, there are usually several days, weeks or sometimes months between the diagnosis and the operation. A patient finds out that a heart valve is no longer fully functioning, so they will have to get a new one in the near or distant future; an aneurysm has been discovered but it is still small, and it is uncertain how it will develop. The preparatory conversation will take a different course if the patients have had time to thoroughly think about their questions, whereas the sudden confrontation with the necessity of an operation comes as a shock.

In emergencies I am especially attentive, as patients are usually so busy with processing their shock that they can absorb only a limited amount of information. I ask if they have really understood everything and try to find out which questions they would ask if they could. I am not on overly slippery terrain when I do this as I have had many such conversations, but I prefer it when we have more time, and the patients can take their time to get used to the idea that they have to have heart surgery. When I find out what makes my patients tick, I can try humor. Some patients display a sort of gallows humor of their own accord. I remember a patient who came to us with a torn aorta. I met him in the emergency department. As always, I sought physical contact; that is important to me. I put my hand on his arm and introduced myself. He knew what was imminent.

"Can you even do that?", he asked. Even though he was in a really bad situation, you could see the mischief in his eyes.

I played along: "I hope so."

"So, you've done this operation before?", he went on.

"Yes, a few times", I replied.

"You are no longer in training?"

"You could say that, yes."

The patient nodded and asked the nurse as if he would no longer trust me: "Is he good, this doctor?"

"You could not be in better hands", my colleague praised me.

"Yes, I believe that, too", he declared. "A heart surgeon without humor can't do a good operation."

The nurse smiled at him encouragingly. "You are really lucky that Dr Natour is on duty tonight."

"Yes, I timed it like this specifically", the patient asserted.

What may sound very flippant here was the patient's testing me to see if he could trust me, even though he was unaware. With other patients I would never have spoken in such a jocular manner; they may have required me to talk about my long experience. In emergency situations like these, when it is essential to gain the patients' trust, it is enormously important to "gain access" to them quickly, just as we will soon "access" them in the operating room to send them into the land of dreams.

I have to admit that in tense situations I have very rarely heard a casual tone like what I just described. Personally, I believe that not only heart surgeons need humor. Humor makes it easier to bear things. Should you have started with your checklist, this would be an item for it: don't lose your sense of humor! And another one: find specialists! Of course, you can listen to the advice of your best friend or you mother-in-law when you have trouble with your relationship or your finances – but you would most likely be better off with a therapist or a financial advisor.

We know from many situations in life that crises may sneak upon you slowly. It may start with a suspicion; later when "by accident" one stumbles upon an explicit message on one's partner's cellphone comes the diagnosis: "My wife has a lover." And finally, the operation, in this case a break-up – ideally with surgical precision and no complications or painful aftermath. The same applies to financial crises, when someone announces the "diagnosis" of insolvency; he is as ruined as the smoking remains of one's house which burned down because a neighbor fell asleep with a burning cigarette.

In medicine there is often a lingering hope that it is all a mistake – after all one sometimes reads about mixed-up lab reports. According to the severity of the discomfort, the patient guesses or knows deep inside that such an assumption is only a vague hope which is rarely confirmed. I have never called off an operation because the diagnosis turned out to be false. Some operations don't happen because sadly the patient dies shortly beforehand. This happens with emergencies but also with people whose heart is severely ill and who may even be waiting for a donor's heart.

In hindsight, many patients who were completely shocked by their diagnosis and certainly had not expected an emergency operation, are happy that they had so little time to deal extensively with what was about to happen. Everything has advantages and disadvantages. Of course, one can prepare better with a scheduled operation: there are many things to put in order if one is going to be away from home for some time (after heart surgery, patients are usually offered rehabilitation). On the other hand, many fears can arise in this time frame. The patients know that they will face a dangerous operation during which many things can go wrong, even though it may have been deemed a routine procedure. It is hard to comprehend the idea that one's heart will be shut down: "Will it start up again? Will there be subsequent damage? Will I be able to still have sex afterwards? Will I be allowed to fly on a vacation with my pacemaker? Will I be able to go with my grandchild to their first day at school?"

Many topics can be discussed and – for the time being – satisfactorily explained during a conversation before the operation. Once the patients come home, however, doubts and new questions may hit them which we will have to address in a second conversation.

The "scheduled" patient will have received and processed a lot of important information about their illness in the past. I am the end of the line, the swing door to the operation. Some patients come to me with a long list of questions. I was once talking to a car salesperson and heard to my surprise that there isn't a great difference between making decisions about a new car or about a heart operation. Some dither, being unsure and hesitant; others make short work of it...if they can afford it (my informant was working for Ferrari).

Even though I may have a lot on my mind, I devote myself to my patients and their relatives during such conversations. I really switch off everything and try to appreciate and get to know the people before me with all my senses. As they will, too. It is a little as if we were dancing around each other, cautiously warming up to each other. If one of my children or my wife calls during a conversation, I take the call. I keep it brief but show my patients that I let them partake in my life, too, that I am a human being like them, made of flesh and blood, not a demigod in white but a doctor to whom they can talk normally.

I can't know why a patient finally gives me their trust – but I can offer them a few things to make it happen. We are both facing a big adventure. It is my aim for the patient to go to the operation with a good feeling, despite all their worries and fears. I want them to trust me. And when that happens, I have the feeling from the first moment of the operation that this body before me, this skin I will cut with a scalpel, this pericardium I will open, and this heart I will hold in my hand, is saying Yes. That is a good feeling for me, and I have confidence in this body, this circulation, this heart; I trust that this heart will travel on this difficult path with me and our team. Together we are strong.

Some patients want to hear specific figures in the preoperative conversation: "What percentage of such operations are successful? What are my chances?" Others avoid this and would rather hear what we say to children: Everything will be fine. And then: kiss it better, mommy.

I cannot answer the most burning question which is usually not asked directly with one hundred percent certainty: will it end well?

We all give our best, but we are only actors, and the direction is out of our hands. The patients, however, put their life in the hands of me and my team. Their life is in acute danger. Then again, no one can really know that, and I aware that there are various possible endings.

There are patients who want to know as little as possible about the details of the operation. "Just do it, you are the specialist."

What may be intended to appear detached is in truth due to their fear, which would increase enormously if they had to deal with the operation in more depth. Other patients have to know everything down to the smallest detail before they agree to the operation: how exactly is the heart-lung machine connected, which thread will be used for sutures and so on. For some patients it is difficult to hand over control. On the stainless-steel table, they will lie under anesthetic, their heart will be shut down, they will be utterly helpless. This feeling is exacerbated by the sheer unavoidability of their situation. They have no other choice, or else the choice would be death.

No two human beings, no two patients are the same. This is obvious from the first meeting to the good-bye when the patients leave the clinic. Some of them visit us occasionally to show us their progress, while from others we don't ever hear again – they are happy to forget us.

One aspect of building trust with patients is to recognize these differences as early as possible. An optimist wants different explanations than a pessimist. A stickler for detail needs different information than a friend of summaries. Someone whose motivation is to achieve something needs to establish different goals than someone who is motivated by leaving something behind: "You will be able to breathe much better again" as opposed to "The pain will go away." There are countless communication details we can pay attention to. The most important thing, however, is to establish a connection to the patient's heart; this will succeed only if I am fully present. Then it will be more than a conversation between doctor and patient, namely a heart-to-heart encounter. In this way I can also feel what drives my patients. Some people like to expose themselves to fear-provoking stimuli because they want to control them. Others would rather avoid them. Every person establishes coping mechanisms in their lives. Some are healthier than others, but a person in a crisis automatically resorts to what they know. If one wants to show them a different path, it will need to happen gently.

In my experience, young people ask less questions during a preoperative conversation. They find it easier to trust, and they are more readily convinced that everything will be okay again. Older people have more experience and know that sometimes things go wrong. You are considered a young patient in heart surgery up to the age of sixty-five. So, a fifty-year-old in need of a new heart valve or a bypass is young for us. And young people, as we know, have little time. They try to negotiate and tell me why they can't have an operation now:

But I wanted to try parachuting again.

My wife is expecting our third child.

Next year would be better.

I have my own business and have to deal with a big assignment.

I have a new job and I am afraid to lose it.

At the start, patients very often see an operation as conflicting with their professional lives. They can't yet fathom how soon that will fade into the background. Indeed, most patients – especially those who define themselves through their job – experience that there is something else, something more important...something without which they would no longer even do their job. Some may even ask themselves something that was unthinkable until now: "Do I even want to continue in this job?" Anyway, this is still far away now, they are at the beginning of a long road. Crises change us. He or she who comes out of a crisis is a different person from the one who entered it. I often wonder why we resist that – after all, nothing helps humans grow quite as much as crises...and love. That is not just a calendar motto – it's the truth.

Differential Diagnosis

There are cases when a patient has come to terms with a diagnosis – and then a second one arrives. Medicine is not infrequently like poking around in the fog. With emergencies particularly it is often not clear what we are facing. Occasionally when we are told to expect a heart attack, it turns out to be a torn aorta. Emergencies are a race against time as every minute counts with some diagnoses. We try to determine what the issue is under the highest pressure. With such cases I am rarely at the frontline; I am second in line. The patients they send me have already been examined by a cardiologist. The colleague calls me: "I have a patient here, possible heart attack. I can see three narrowed vessels in the heart catheter. Looking at the tissue, I don't think I could place a stent. Do you have time for three bypasses?"

There are clearly defined rules as to when a stent is placed and when it's a bypass. A CT scan or echocardiography can help with the decision, but it will only become clear what one is up against once the operation is underway. Every tissue is different, but *how* different is something I can neither see nor sense. The vessel wall may be calcified or fragile, which impedes suture.

The decision about how to proceed is made by the whole heart team, with the colleagues from the left and right sides of the corridor coming together like two ventricles of a heart. And then we will do the best for the patient. If the aorta is torn, we will operate immediately, as every minute counts.

According to statistics, seven minutes pass until a doctor arrives after an emergency call in Germany; numbers for the USA and the UK are similar. What a superb safety net for people! However, once an unlucky person is trapped in this net and their identity changes from person to patient, our society does not appear quite as helpful anymore.

Sometimes I become furious when I hear that someone is afraid to lose their job because of an operation. No employer should be allowed to threaten this, not even subtly; reality, however, looks different. If you show a weakness, things may become hard for you later along the lines of: we can't rely on this employee, he's constantly sick, potentially unstable...he can't be promoted. Strangely this overlooks the fact that an employee who has successfully mastered a serious crisis has considerably improved his skill set. It is a little bit like the case of working mothers. Everyone knows they can be multitasking, socially competent, team-minded top managers with enormous innovative capacity and other valuable qualities – and yet they don't get the fabulous jobs as their child might be sick occasionally. And what happens then? Well, the competent top manager will find a way – and society should finally find it, too. The Netherlands is ahead in this regard.

The pressure to function, and the fear of falling through the cracks of our performance society because one needs heart surgery, are ingrained in many people, and cause them great grief. This can even lead to the affected person developing a guilty conscience towards their families or employers or even their health insurance.

Most of the time, a relative or friend accompanies the patient to a preoperative conversation. I like this and think it's important, because four ears hear more than two and one can compare notes afterwards. The trust of the relatives is nearly as important to me as the trust of my patients. Of course, they will compare notes to see if they can really trust this surgeon. I want for my patients to have a good feeling after the conversation. They should know that I am a very experienced surgeon who will look after them well. Many of them would have checked up on me and read testimonials on the internet. When I realize that recommendations from others are important to them, I tell them that in the Netherlands I am a surgeon with the best rating and give them the link. Digital natives can feel it click, and I'm in.

Dr. Google

During my training, doctors still had the final say when it came to a diagnosis. They were the undisputed specialists. Today we fight against Dr. Google, who is all-knowing – and this is exactly how some patients arrive for their consultation. I have colleagues whose blood pressure rises when a sentence starts with "I read on the internet that…"

I find it brilliant that people can gather so much information today so easily. I am also a great friend of patient forums. I want to establish a dialogue between patients and experts, for the benefit of both, through my own foundation. Often, however, Dr. Google serves as an accelerator of fear. You notice that when you just google "sniffles". Is it just the sniffles or rather a life-threatening infection with COVID-19? I like it when patients investigate their illness, but I also tell them something that applies nearly always: "what your neighbor has or Dr. Google's patient or someone from a patient forum has, is not the same as what you have." I offer them evidence which can't be easily dismissed: "I have operated on countless patients with the same diagnosis, but for every one of them the baseline is different, the pre-existing conditions, the circumstances and also the quality of the tissue. So, if you want my opinion: Dr. Google is a superb theorist, but I would not let him operate on me."

8

PATIENT
JARGON

As a young doctor during an internship, I had an experienced colleague who did not want to promise his patients too much. He pointed out the dangers in every sentence. He was the type that always played it safe. It took him months to buy a new car because he scrutinized everything. Once I was a witness to a conversation, he had with one of his patients. He eyed the young woman before him with a frown and then sighed: "You know, this is an extremely difficult operation."

What was this man saying? I would have liked to cut him off. Of course, we weren't talking about taking out an appendix here, but my idea of "extremely difficult" was different from his. We were talking about implanting a heart valve, as hers had been impaired, presumably the result of a neglected cold. We call this endocarditis, an inflammation of the myocardium caused by viruses or bacteria.

The patient nodded sorrowfully.

"It is possible that one does not survive it", my colleague continued. At least he had not said "you can die". I was too young back then to clearly convey my thoughts to my older colleague, but I tried – sadly without success. He shrugged his shoulders and said that every doctor has their methods, and that I would no longer nurture false hopes for my patients once I had been in the job for a longer time.

Today I think he was a hopeless case. I did not want to nurture false hopes but put fears to rest. Patients are afraid before an operation in any case. We should focus on things that give them strength, without sugarcoating matters. Even though I will be very honest and tell my patients clearly that they will experience losses after a heart operation, we can focus on their new quality of life. I will definitely not foster doubt in my patients about the abilities of the operation team, but radiate confidence to convey that we have things under control. To show you how much I'm in control, I will share one of my favorite jokes:

The patient is wheeled into the operating room. The surgeon leans over him and says: "Everything's fine, David." He nods encouragingly. "All will be well, never fear, David, all will be well." He nods again, then continues: "It will all be alright, David, you'll manage." The patient who had tried to speak a few times is now very unnerved. He interrupts the surgeon tentatively: "But my name is not David, doctor." The surgeon nods again. "I know. I am called David."

All of us know people who spend a lot of time worrying unnecessarily, while others would never do that: Under no circumstances do I need an overdose of horror scenarios, keep them away from me! One such person was Mr. Huber. Okay, his arm had hurt here and there, but blame it on the work in the garden. He just wasn't the type to suffer a heart attack, had always been healthy, three minutes under the cold shower every morning, and never white bread, only whole wheat. No, he hadn't gone to a doctor's practice because only malingerers hang out there. Of course, Mr. Huber needed a different approach than Mrs. Bauer who (in Mr. Huber's opinion) was one such malingerer. She can hear the grass grow and now feels reassured because a tumor was found early through her sensitivity. With Mr. Huber, a tumor could have grown to the size of a water polo ball before he may have had the vague suspicion that something may not be right. Isn't it fascinating how different people can be? How much about themselves they reveal to me as their doctor, thereby showing which kind of support may be good for them during therapy and would be in harmony with their coping strategy for their crisis. To apply therapy against a patient's will is usually futile. But – attention, checklist! – we should become conscious of our thought patterns. Some kinds of resistance we keep up only out of sheer habit. We might get in our own way during a crisis and can even stumble over our own dogmas – which in the worst case can be fatal.

Diagnosis: Dogma

A crisis causes a state of emergency. We must think differently than usual because we will act differently. Every dogma we defend, every opinion we insist on can turn the crisis into a disaster. "I've always been in good health" is one such dogma, as is "chemicals make you sick, and I won't take any tablets." Or: "I've always exercised, never smoked, hence nothing can happen to me."

As we often don't know the origin of our dogmas, we must make absolutely sure we don't get fooled by them. The words *as a matter of principle* provide a good hint here: "I don't think much of doctors as a matter of principle." Yes, a doctor needs to be able to deal with something like that – and we should use the chance to convince a patient otherwise!

In the end it is about our locus of control, to use a psychological term. Are we ourselves responsible for our calamity, or is it a powerful "other", or bad luck, or fate? How we answer this also depends on the specific matter at hand. A patient who should lose weight urgently can blame his wife: she cooks so well, so I just can't help it. Or they have heavy bones, for which their parents and genes are responsible. Or they burn calories slowly and thus gain weight, which is not their fault either. Or they simply have the bad luck they always have. In any case, they just can't help it.

But the thing is, the larger a person is, the higher is the risk during an operation. It starts with the way access to the operating field can be impeded. Other risks include longer operating times, potentially with heavier loss of blood. On top of that, there are often obesity-associated conditions such as high blood pressure, diabetes or sleep apnea. The regulation of blood pressure and blood sugar will be more difficult for such patients, and their mobilization slower. This may entail postoperative complications such as wound healing disorders, decubitus, thromboses and infections.

We put such patients on a diet by using diplomacy, as we know that if they like to shift responsibility to others, they will have to "follow" the doctor who proposes a dietary change. Why don't you test yourself: do you think that others, circumstances, or fate are to blame if something doesn't work the way you'd want, and you're unable to do something about it? Or do you believe you have a say, too? And isn't it fascinating to notice how some things you think are carved in stone are changeable – while other matters you thought were pliable are nonnegotiable? In conversations with former patients, I have often heard how surprised they were when they discovered new things about themselves. A woman once put it very nicely: "The heavy time I had to get through made me lighter."

Often, we judge ourselves much more harshly than others, whom we readily allow some weaknesses. A severe illness is not a minor weakness but a major debility which can last for a long time. However much a patient may try, they won't be able to act like they are used to. This realization is hard to digest, especially for strong-willed people who are convinced that their success is exclusively in their hands. After having been bedridden for quite some time, they want to get up and find they can't. Their legs won't support them anymore. After brushing their teeth, they are so tired they must sleep. They are not familiar with such things and can now no longer recognize themselves. Up until now they were their body's boss. When the body seizes control, a human being becomes very small – and suddenly we are in the realm of philosophy: is the human being the same as their body? Everyone will have their own answer, which is fine if it does not become a dogma.

If I had applied the same approach to Mrs. Bauer and Mr. Huber, I would have overlooked something essential. If they had the same indication, they would obviously undergo the same operation – which would, however, look very differently for them. Mrs. Bauer's open thorax looks different than Mr. Huber's; and yet differences do not play a role in the kind of medicine which is geared towards functionality and economic feasibility. In my opinion, that is a disastrous mistake. If I take different approaches to Mrs. Bauer and Mr. Huber – in our preoperative conversations, during the postoperative care, in rehabilitation and later – the health insurance will probably save a lot of money and, in the end, time. What does one have to expend to achieve this? Something priceless – something which is very simple and very complicated at the same time.

Before the Cut: Listen

Listening is becoming more and more of an art in our society – and this art is constantly disappearing. Medicine is no exception here. We are in danger of forgetting how to listen if we rely nearly always on machines to diagnose people. The patient becomes an object with sockets, so to speak, into which we plug our medical high tech:

Where is the USB port? The catheter for a patient of this age into the groin, please. We look at the screen. The patient's saying something... Why haven't we managed to delete the audio from the patient-object? Being human, how annoying! And how he hems and haws, looks for words, describes something utterly irrelevant...oh hurry up! And why does he have to say anything at all, it's all very clear, I can see what's wrong with him, it's bleeding obvious. No need to hem and haw or waste time.

Really?

What about an indication that does not fit the patient's condition? Both nouns come with the suffix –tion but are very different. "You're bound for the wheelchair with this lumbar spine", a charming orthopedist once said to a school friend of mine. She is a belly dancer, laughed in his face and snaked out of his office.

"It's not possible that you're in pain", my neighbor heard from a gastroenterologist after a gastroscopy. "There's nothing there." Many patients with chronic pain suffer double when there is no medical explanation for their pain – which does not mean that they are only imagining it. A doctor who only wants to believe what can be measured may think such a patient a malingerer. I find this odd, especially in a time when our technical possibilities enable us to know that we are surrounded by invisible things – have you ever seen a coronavirus, I mean in the wild rather than on TV?

Doctors look through microscopes, but who says that there isn't another way to look at things? Well, sometimes one has to listen in order to see. To see with one's ears – in my mind, that is part of a doctor's art. Even when an indication displayed by a monitor fits a patient's condition, I can gather further important information by listening to them. Most importantly, in this way I can find out how best to help this specific patient, because I get to know them a bit and develop an individual plan for them, which details the best therapy and care. That is exactly what I love about my profession. I want to help people reclaim some of their quality of life, and as I like to be successful, I choose the direct path to my goal: to include the whole human being rather than just their current problem.

When we focus exclusively on computer screens and evaluate reconstructions in 3D or 4D, however, we miss the whole human being. Focusing on the visible, we miss the track to the invisible where a solution may lie. Listening is hard work; one must attend to the patient thoroughly. I can process many images at the same time but can't follow more than one conversation. To listen to a patient means that in this moment they are the most important thing and I attend to them with all my senses. How do they look...sick? I sense their mental state. I feel their hand, moist or cold. I hear their voice...are they resigned, afraid, calm? Sometimes I can smell their fear. I listen to them with my whole being, and they sense that I am there for them, and the doors to their innermost being open one by one, like heart valves. Suddenly they tell me something seemingly unrelated to the diagnosis, and yet their subconscious has sent me a signal: "That is important, you have to tell the doctor." Maybe it is the wings of a soul which have opened rather than the valves of a heart.

"There was this sharp, shooting pain in my chest two or three years ago. I felt nauseous after that, didn't feel well. It was during a ski trip. Maybe I had overdone it a bit, but my wife was far ahead of me, and I didn't want to lag behind. Strange that I remember that now, I had forgotten it completely."

"Did you tell your wife back then?"

"No, I told no one. I didn't want to be seen as weak."

I did not only get important medical information here, presumably about a silent heart attack, but also learned something about the patient: he finds it hard to show weakness. I will make sure to appeal to the strength in him. I will not say: "You will have to get used to this lack of strength", but rather: "Once you have all this behind you, you will properly regain your strength."

And I will pass all this on to my team.

Medical professionals of course know that communication with their patients is important. They may attend a course teaching constructive conversation skills, a voluntary additional training which is not an obligatory part of their medical degree course. That is most laudable, but when the certificate of participation is the end of it, it is no more than another unused skill. Communication with the patients should, in my opinion, be an integral part of medical training: how do I talk to them, how do I gain their trust, how do I react when confronted with their emotional reactions such as despair, fear, tears...or when they become impolite due to stress? How do I come to terms with people's severe misfortunes? All this should ideally be practiced in role plays so doctors can experience closely for themselves what it is like to be confronted with a terrible diagnosis and how it feels to feel helpless in the face of a seemingly all-knowing doctor. These role plays should be repeated, just like pilots are asked to practice in a simulator in regular intervals. Effective communication with the patients must become second nature for doctors, just like the use of a stethoscope. One aim of our foundation *Stilgezet* is to instigate such changes. We advocate for young medical professionals to develop good communication skills. If you have another look at the graph (above at the end of the chapter OPENING), you will understand how important communication is for each of the stages. In uncertain situations, communication builds bridges onto solid ground. Patients must have the right to ask and get answers, within an appropriate time frame. All this should not be an appendix to medical training but form the basis for the patients' trust – whose recovery in turn is accelerated as they feel well cared for. Trust and the reduction of stress foster health, while fear and stress harm it.

I want to motivate medical professionals to have the courage to be human when wearing a white coat, to meet other people when they're in dire straits – without it affecting us so much that we can no longer act professionally. Yes, this is a fine line, but in the end, I am convinced that it is more fulfilling for both patients and doctors. Medical training at university and all other medical courses should teach how we can achieve this and manage this fine line.

I am not a psychologist. I don't believe it's necessary to be one to get in touch with the patients. It is about taking the time to listen and open one's own heart to people who are in a dire situation; life experience will do the rest. In my opinion, it is a mistake to assume a good doctor is not meant to show they have a heart – and it's sad, too. We do not need to be afraid of each other, not the patients of the doctors nor the doctors of the patients. Even so, it sometimes seems to me as if patients and doctors circle each other like opponents. In part this is owing to the exaggerated reverence towards the medical profession in Germany. In the Netherlands, the hierarchies are less pronounced. I would like for us to play in a team everywhere, with each other instead of against. Professionalism and compassion are not mutually exclusive. Compassion does not obscure reason, whereas pity does. If I exercise compassion, I remain a doctor – and according to my definition, a better one.

In the everyday proceedings of a clinic, it is hard to find time for such encounters. But they will happen if one really wants it to, for the good of everyone involved: the patients, staff, and in the end, the clinic's financial statements, too. If we listen, double examinations are eliminated, and we can save a lot of money and avoid false diagnoses. For that to happen, however, we must be in the here and now in our contact with patients. What a patient tells me is ephemeral; they say something – and often I must interpret what they really mean. Are they the kind who would rank the pain someone else would call a ten as a five?

I can always look again at an indication or image later, as many times as I wish – but I cannot ask it questions and go into detail, whereas I can ask my patients to provide more specific information.

With an image that poses a question, I will need a further examination, another imaging procedure. We tend to reduce our perception more and more to things that are visible, as if only they could convey the truth.

Listening will ultimately also help us if complications occur during treatment. What would this person have wanted? We can only answer that if we get to know them – as human beings, not as cases.

Why is listening not taught? What is unpleasant about it? Have we forgotten how to be human? Or are we approaching it all wrong? Why are we drifting apart from each other, even though closeness would improve outcomes? Is it sometimes because there isn't an answer to everything, that we have no reply to some questions from patients? How can we teach this perspective to young doctors who have grown up as digital natives and from whom we older ones in turn can also learn a lot?

Before the Click: Caring Affection

A new generation of medical professionals is evolving which has grown up with high-tech medicine. They have a closer relationship with their equipment than with their patients, whom they sometimes find outright irritating. High-tech medicine knows thresholds, percentages, charts – but treating patients is not merely about finding the strategy best suited to the machines, but the one that suits the individual patient. What that might be, we can find out as medical professionals by an interdisciplinary approach and by turning towards the patient. We must not make the mistake of forgetting the human being in our enthusiasm about our technical possibilities.

Listening and caring affection go hand in hand. *I care about you; I'm listening to you.* I am not putting emphasis on this to show what a wonderful doctor I am because I hold my patients' hands. I'm writing this to tell you how these encounters which focus on the patients' well-being touch my heart as well.

Apart from this, there is also a clear medical reason for me to touch my patients' feet, too, when I visit them in intensive care. After an operation, a person is in a critical condition. All vessels are narrowed because we had to cool down their blood. In the meantime, we warmed it up again, and the vessels widen; a blood volume shift to the periphery may lead to a critical situation.

I became a doctor because I wanted to work with people, not just machines – and I definitely do not want to treat people like machines. I want to pass on my own enjoyment of the medical profession. In case you're not a doctor: when you get the chance, ask your physician why they chose their profession – it doesn't always have to be the medicine woman or man who starts a personal conversation. What's the point of this strange, stiff respect? One room, two people, one affliction. Go on, dare… to hearken, too!

"Hearken" is a word well suited to the heart. One hearkens to one's heart. Maybe we should make a habit of it: to hearken more, into ourselves and around ourselves. The heart even has ears. That is the name for the excrescences of the atria which look like two big ears. They are what makes the heart, heart-shaped. During an operation concerning atrial fibrillation the heart ears are closed off from the inside with stitches, because otherwise dangerous blood clots may occur. Sometimes they are even cut off because we believe that many of the nerve tracts involved in the atrial fibrillation run inside the ears. As far as my patients are concerned, I notice that they are often more clairaudient after an operation than before. In any case, they have a different relationship with their heart than people whose heart has never seen the light of a surgical lamp.

Presumably you have consulted a few doctors in your life. Which ones do you remember, and why? The one who was so quick to operate their computer? I suspect you will remember those doctors who showed you loving care, listened to you, made you feel you're in good hands with them. Am I right?

Some doctors you will not be able to remember, even though they saved your life, for example in intensive care. The doctors there who are fighting for human lives often have no personal contact with their patients as they are in a coma or are unable to remember anything once they leave intensive care.

But the fact remains: We all can shape every encounter according to our convictions. Sure, that requires from us doctors a high degree of attentiveness in order not to slide into our automatic mode, switching on the autopilot and focusing more on our technical devices' helpers than our patients. Countless studies have shown that the healing process partly depends on how caring we act towards a patient. Caring also means that we do not merely offer services covered by a patient's health insurance – possible at the cheapest rates – but add specific human help.

A human being touches another person because they care for them out of love or benevolence. Parents, children, lovers, relatives, friends. If a stranger touches us on exposed parts of our body, we are usually standing in front of a doctor or a physiotherapist. In a way a border is crossed here, but it is legal. The border crossing may open the gate to the soul, too. Unfortunately, less and less doctors examine their patients with their hands – and yet that was once normal and part of the first contact. I believe I must be more and more careful not to insist on an old normal – but it is dear to my heart that it is not forgotten. I recently overheard a conversation between two women by accident. Torn between consternation and astonishment, the first told the second that her new doctor had touched her: "Properly, with her hands on my tummy and tapping my knee with a reflex hammer."

"I want to go see her, too", the other one said and took out her cellphone to note down the doctor's name.

The fact that we deem it worth mentioning to be

touched by a doctor is rather sad. Nevertheless, I had to smile when I heard those women talk about it.

I know from my own experience how thankful patients are even when I touch their arm only fleetingly: "Did you sleep well?", or when I look at a wound and briefly touch the affected area. This touch is not important for the healing, but it gives the patient a good feeling and strengthens them in their struggle towards recovery. They are perceived as human beings – even though they may lie in a bed at that moment and may deem themselves worthless. Someone turns to them caringly, and nothing is expected of them in exchange.

I do not plead for a return to the era of the ear trumpet...but maybe the stethoscope? That, after all, is how you used to recognize a doctor; today, however, a stethoscope is a necklace rather than a medical instrument. A stethoscope, a word whose meaning in Greek is *chest monitor*, is a very important non-invasive instrument which can capture valve noises and certain sounds in the lungs very well. The stethoscope should be the instrument we apply first, not the x-ray machine.

To use a stethoscope does not mean to forego ultrasound, but it simply offers the opportunity to establish physical contact – maybe like a handshake (which will probably go out of fashion due to COVID). As a surgeon, I am surrounded by high tech and without it would not be able to work. But technology should not always be our first choice. How often do patients come to a physician's office and are x-rayed before they have even seen the doctor – "so that the doc can get a picture of your condition".

No, the doc does not *get* a picture, he *has one done*.

A patient told me of an appointment with a doctor. He

wanted a consultation about the arrhythmia of his wife, who refused to go to the doctor herself. The assistant sent the substitute patient straight to the ECG. "But nothing's wrong with me", he said. "You can't possibly know that", she countered and explained than an ECG would have to be done routinely before that patient was allowed to see the doctor. Upon this, the patient was so confused – *is that so, and what if something turns out to be wrong with me, but I'm here because of my wife* – that when he finally spoke with the doctor, who gave the impression he was pressed for time, the patient could only put forth a fraction of his concerns.

Here is another story, probably an even stranger one. An acquaintance told me about her examination at a proctologist. She was led to a cool examination room full of high tech, which she described as a space capsule. An assistant handed her paper underpants with a hole. She put it on and then waited shivering for twenty-five minutes for the doctor, dressed in her horrible lingerie. When the doctor came in, he did not even look at her but went straight to his computer and started typing something.

"Why did you put up with it for so long?", I asked.

"Because I was glad to have managed to get the appointment."

"Did no one there ask you why you were there?", I inquired.

"On the phone I had told them I may have hemorrhoids."

I imagined for a patient of mine to say to me: "Doctor, I may have a heart attack", upon which we cut them open – and when we sew them up again it has turned out to only have been lovesickness. Okay, lovesickness can hurt a lot, but does it require heart surgery? That's only possible if the patient has private health insurance – please indulge my little joke.

My acquaintance left the doctor's office with good advice from the assistant, who had defended her boss, and with the words "The doctor has been working since 8am without a break" scotched any suggestion for improvement. The good advice was that, as the doctor hadn't found anything wrong, she should try psyllium.

"And?"

"Great tip. It helped." She grinned. "Next time I will speak to the assistant first. That will save money, as such an examination is expensive."

"Speak to the doctor anyway", I told her. "Sometimes we are running in the rat race morning to night and don't notice how we have lost our own focus – and our focus towards our patients."

Who or what is to blame? It is easy to write "the system" – and yet I am convinced that is true, as I believe we are entering a dead-end street, and at such high speed that hardly anyone has time to ponder. In his book *Den kranken Menschen verstehen* [Understanding the Sick Human Being], medical ethicist and philosopher Giovanni Maio exposes many shortcomings and advocates a medicine of loving care. Like him, I believe that we don't only need a few individuals who propose alternatives, but many patients and doctors who desire a medicine for the human being. In this "medicine of loving care", as Maio calls it, we are aware of the fact that there are severe crises in life. We should fight less against death than for quality of life, and we know that the aim is not to reach the old normal after an illness but to shape a new normal. I would like for us to make the transition soon!

In gynecology, we see mothers-to-be who stare at a monitor and watch their baby like they watch TV, instead of listening inward. Their contact with the unborn child in their uterus is primarily visual; this is also due to the intensive medical supervision of pregnancies, which today are treated like an illness in some places: giving birth seems to have become impossible without medical assistance.

And the same applies to dying. More and more people die in the hospital. I observe that relatives, too, partly orient themselves less by the condition of their loved ones, but rather by the monitors above the bed. Instead of holding a hand, talking, stroking, they stare at monitors and call the nurses: "The number was above a hundred just then, now it is above." "The red line keeps jumping and there's a beep. Is that dangerous?"

Yes, there's a beep. And yes, that is dangerous.

9

CONVALESCENCE

My first patient one particular afternoon was not so young anymore, sixty-five years old, and was to get a bypass. Two days ago, during a heart catheter examination, our cardiologist had found that it would not be possible to use a stent. But Mr. Braun did not want to accept the necessity of an operation "just because I have private health insurance"; on top of this a work colleague had got a stent last year. "You don't notice anything, he's back to his old self." Calmly I explained to the patient that in his case a long-term prognosis with stents was not good. But he absolutely did not want an operation. His wife seemed outright desperate. I could tell that she had beseeched her husband in the last forty-eight hours to agree to the bypass...to no avail.

What a patient's relatives must bear in this phase is sometimes almost superhuman. Another word for relatives is "dependents", and it is very fitting: I depend on another, in good times and bad. Hereafter I mention a few thoughts about this connection which can be infinitely helpful but also destructive:

If you're well, I'm well too.

    If you're feeling bad, I'm not well either.

    If you're not well but pretend you are, I'm feeling bad and will try to help you admit that you're not well.

    Why do you not let me share your affliction?

    A problem shared is a problem halved.

    Do you think I'm too weak for your worries?

    Why do you say everything's fine, why don't you admit that nothing, nothing, nothing is fine?

    I'm not allowed to say anything, as otherwise you get upset.

    I have to pretend everything's fine.

    Because you make the rules.

    But you're bluffing.

    I'm losing my mind because you do none of the things the doctor told you to do.

    I don't want to remind you constantly about your tablets.

    You are an adult, but you behave like a little toddler.

    I feel as if I'm bound and gagged.

    You're driving me away from you.

    You don't have to pretend you're strong.

    If you do that, I can't feel you.

    Let us get through this together.

I would so much like to be there for you. Especially now.

Please, don't be so dismissive.

I can't bear to see you suffer.
It breaks my heart.
How oh how can I help you?

I don't want for everything to change.
I simply do not want it!

If you had smoked less and lived more healthily as I always told you, you would not be in this situation now. And then once you're in the clinic, who will have to take care of everything? And later?
You are inconsiderate. But I must not tell you that.
I have to be really nice. Otherwise, you'll think me evil.

Will you now become an old and sick man?
I feel young. I want to live!

How long will this go on for?
All this waiting drives me crazy.
When will we finally get a date for the operation?
I am so afraid, and don't want you to notice.
I wake up at night and hear you breathe and think what would it be like if there was suddenly silence beside me...
Forever...

To Unburden One's Heart

When a person gets a terrible diagnosis, not only his relatives will sometimes be unable to recognize them –

they may become a stranger to themselves. Without wanting to, out of deep despair which they can't share, they rebuff those around them who want to support them. They acquire an armor and appear unapproachable, adversarial. Relatives and friends often only understand later that these are protective mechanisms.

Some ill people harbor thoughts they are ashamed of. For example, they may hate others for the fact that they are in good health. Yet at the same time, they are those the patients love most in life, and they would never wish them ill...at least it was like this when everything was still normal.

It is enormously important to see through these mechanisms, for one day there will be a new normal which will grow out of our behavior during this crisis. We are the result of our past. We shape our tomorrow today.

The relatives' reaction to rejection, abrasiveness, insults etc. will depend on the extent of their psychological insight or simply on the maturity of their personality. If they take everything personally and let themselves be drawn into superficial dramas, the situation can escalate. Someone needs to take the lead, ideally one of the healthy relatives. But when it is the person who is usually in authority who falls ill, they may well want to hold on to it. More than that, they may feel they *must* remain in authority, as otherwise they might feel even more confused and worthless. By doing this, however, they deprive themselves of the relief they could experience if they were to signal to the others: let me rest for a while. And the others could say: sure, we'll do that, we'll stand in for you until you have recovered.

When I notice that a family's situation threatens to get out of hand, I sometimes try to moderate. Usually, I recommend psychological support. In my opinion, this should be provided to patients and their relatives as a matter of course, as crutches are to someone with a broken leg. There are prehistories which make failures very likely, for example when a successful man who has handed his family life over to his wife completely and was more like a guest at his own home, falls ill soon after his retirement. He thereby breaks the agreement that "once he is finally free" they would now follow the wife's interests – opening a boarding kennel, take a trip around the world, move to the country or whatever else it may be. The wife had held back for many years. But now none of her wishes will come true, at least not in the way they both had imagined. The clinic instead of the Caribbean. Depending on how deep the love is, which will become clear very quickly in such a case, a lot of bitterness and anger may erupt.

Something always comes up.
        But that's not my fault!
        But of course, it is! If only you...

Recriminations and feelings of guilt weigh down heavily on people who are already battered. From experience I know that frankness is the best way to proceed here: they should talk to each other – disburden their hearts to each other, as they say. After all, the hearts of the relatives are full of affliction, too, and they live through the five phases of coming to terms with a crisis (see above) with all the associated emotions.

A crisis or a severe illness can also weld couples,

families, and friends together. They realize how much they love each other; how important they are for one another. They remember what they have experienced together, all the highs and lows. They draw strength from the challenges they have mastered, encourage each other, form new ties with each other in their hearts, stand up for each other. Even people who were a bit distant before will now come very close together. They sense what life is about. Sometimes they are even thankful to have been given this "lesson", as a patient once expressed it. "I am glad all this has happened", she said. "Before it, we had been co-existing rather than living together. My illness showed us how important we are for each other, and what life is all about, namely love and connectedness and the good feelings one shares with each other, even after all these years. We said yes to each other once again and did so deliberately."

Other couples discover things about each other which surprise them. "I would die for my wife", a man once told me in tears. "I had not felt that before. I love her so much, and now I know how much. When she lay there so pale in a coma with all these tubes, it broke my heart."

I heard this from a woman: "I always thought I'm the cool type. We never spoke about feelings at home. We were intellectuals, and proud of it. But when my husband was so severely ill, I did not master it intellectually. For the first time in my life, I felt such a deep readiness to be loving and caring inside me I would never have thought possible."

Another woman discovered an entirely new task for herself: "My husband had always been in charge. Then suddenly he was unable to do that, and I had to take over. That weighed me down at first and I would have liked

WHEN LIFE COMES TO A STANDSTILL   111

to hide in a corner and cry, but that wasn't possible as now it was my turn. So, I did what had to be done, albeit grudgingly as I had not chosen it. But after I while I began to enjoy it, and today we have a relationship on equal terms, which is good for both of us."

We should share such changes for the better with others as they show us that to leave old behavior patterns behind is worth it. To shed our familiar skin, to try something new. When I recount such stories amongst my colleagues, some are surprised: "No one tells me such things."

On one such occasion a colleague retorted: "Because you just wouldn't want to hear them."

Yes, I believe my patients sense that I am interested in them beyond their hearts and their blood vessels. I have told some of them about our foundation. It is important to collect as much information as possible to be able to optimally support people who are at the beginning of a hard road.

There is not always a happy ending, especially if things aren't going well in general and there were many small crises smoldering before the big one. If she could have her way, Mrs. Müller would pack her things and take to her heels. Ever since her brother's birth, she had had nothing but trouble with him. And now this to cap it all off: a heart operation, just when she wanted to get out of this destructive entanglement for good. How often had he lied to her, duped her, even stole from her?

But she is all he has got.

To go now...she does not have the heart to do it.

Or does she?

What will the others think of her?

All they see is the poor brother, as always!

She doesn't even have a choice!

But she does. At least she should have a choice. None of us should be this quick to judge. Sure, one doesn't abandon a vulnerable person. And yes, in a crisis like this people can be reconciled. But we don't know the history here, and we are not entitled to any judgement.

As for most situations, there is also a codex for behavior during an illness. One just does not separate from a partner or abandon a family member during a severe illness. Such expectations put a lot of pressure on those affected. They reproach themselves bitterly when they do not conform to the image of a caring and loving person which society imposes on them in this situation. Someone is sick, someone else is standing by them, gives them strength, and all will be well in the end... and they will live happily ever after.

"Doctor, I believe I am a bad person. My husband is not to blame, but every time he pants in this way when he has trouble breathing...I become really aggressive!"

Of course, I only get to hear such things if we have built a trusting relationship over some time. Sometimes such conversations seem like confessions to me. When I can say: "You are not the first to tell me something like this", people are very relieved.

There are good days and bad days, we are human beings, not saints. We should accept that and not compare ourselves to ideals we can never hope to reach. Where do they come from? If no one talks about the darker side of things, everyone not living up to the ideal will feel inadequate – as if they were the only ones with whom there is something wrong. But that is not true. Therefore I opt for talking about everything as openly as possible, so that people notice: I am not alone after all, others have these feelings, too!

It is part of the relatives' fate that they have a lot to bear before a big operation. They are on the frontline even though they have no physical pain. They are hit with the full extent of the patients' despair and all their extreme emotions. They themselves feel despair (not wanting to let on about it) and fear (which they also keep to themselves). Once a woman told me: "Ultimately, I am even more affected than my husband. If it goes wrong, he will be gone, but he won't notice that – whereas I would have to go on living without him...which I would very much notice."

Such clear words are rarely spoken by patients and relatives; mostly such fear is disguised as worry, or else someone plays the hero...but in the end these are all masquerades of fear. When we fall out of our normal, we are afraid, and from the beginning – it is as simple as that.

How about a checklist at this point? After all, it is the key to smart crisis management.

- – Collect information from different sources.
- – Get a clear picture of your situation.
- – Expose all behavior patterns and dogmas which could impede you.
- – Make yourself aware that the situation is what it is and that it is up to you how it will continue.
- – Find allies with whom you can speak openly.
- – Always listen to your gut feeling.
- – Make yourself aware of your resources: this is probably not the first crisis in your life so you know what you need and how you can mobilize strength.

- – Have courage and be optimistic.
- – You can revise a decision you made at any time.

That is what my patient Mr. Braun did whom I introduced to you at the start of this chapter. Do you remember? He did not want a bypass but a stent, even though the diagnosis advised against it.

"The condition of your vessels suggests a stent would pose too high a risk of complications", I explained to him once again, while his wife nodded sorrowfully, twirling a wet tissue.

"What sort of complications?", he asked gruffly. I had explained that to him already, too, but now the door was open a tiny bit for the first time. Sometimes I ask myself how I can be so patient, as patience is usually not one of my strengths. But when I see a patient's situation through their eyes, it is relatively easy to be patient. In his situation, I would also be glad to have a patient doctor by my side who moves at my speed instead of forcing his own on me.

"A vessel could tear, bleedings would follow…which would result in an emergency operation. I can only repeat myself: in your case, an operation would be best."

Mrs. Braun sighed heavily. She looked at her husband, pleading and angry at the same time.

Mr. Braun said abruptly: "Our grandkids, twins, they like playing soccer best."

"You can still score goals with a bypass", I said. "Not straight after the operation, but after a while."

"Okay", he said then.

Shocked, his wife dropped her tissue which looked like

a collection of many white worms. "I didn't mean to do that", she said, startled.

"I don't know if I can sew those together again", I said. "But I can try."

The three of us laughed. It was a relief.

This is how I met the Brauns, and Mrs. Braun has since sent me a card every Easter and Christmas. In my experience, men and women handle the prospect of an operation differently, both as patients and as relatives. It is a difference in their behavior pattern: men can endure less than women, and sometimes they don't even come along to the appointment because they are afraid. So instead of the patient I will face their wife, who has her best female friend with her for support.

This reminds me of the differences when people give directions. Women remember landmarks. Turn left at the billboard, straight on to the red house, then right. A man stays on the main street and keeps North at the gas station. If I give directions to a woman, I won't send her North, and I won't mention a red house as a clue to a man. Which house? Was there a house? Red? What? It is no use becoming impatient either when the man does not see the house, or when the woman walks in a circle. What *is* useful, though – to bring this back to medical matters – is personalized medicine. That is what we are working on in our clinic, to be able to support each patient and their relatives individually.

I remember a patient who did not want an operation. "My life was beautiful", she said. "It was a fulfilled life. I'm in my mid-seventies now. If you operate on my heart valve, it will take a long time until I'm back on my feet again, and you said yourself that some aspects of my life will be limited."

"Yes. The quality of your life will be considerably lower."

"I do not want that."

You hardly ever meet such clear-thinking patients. This women impressed me a lot. In the end I did operate on her because her husband implored me to. She agreed against her own will, so to speak. Four months after the operation her husband informed me that she had died while walking her dog. He sounded very sad on the phone, and he was aware that she had undertaken the operation for him. Although he was sorry about that, he was infinitely grateful for those final four months. "It was only during this time that I found the strength to go on without her."

"What a farewell present", I said before I could help it.

He, too, sends me an email now and then with a photo of his dog.

A couple of about sixty is also memorable. She handled "the matter" like a tradesperson. The pump is broken, needs to be repaired, then all will run smoothly again. In contrast, the fear was written all over her husband's face.

"As far as I'm concerned, it's all clear, I have no further questions", she announced.

Her husband nodded obediently.

We were done, and the two got up.

Suddenly it all erupted from the man. "I am so afraid that something will go wrong, I am so damn afraid." He covered his face with his hands and began to cry.

I usually know what I will do next; heart surgeons make quick decisions. In this case, however, I decided to do nothing at all. I remained seated and was quiet. The two of them no longer noticed me, and I witnessed a deeply moving scene. The couple stood in a close embrace near the door, and suddenly the patient began to cry, which made the husband regain his composure.

"Sorry", they said together, as if they had rehearsed it. Then they took each other's hand and left.

Later in the elevator I ran into our psychologist and told her about those two. She explained that the husband had taken on his wife's pain as a kind of proxy to protect her from it.

For Love

Wonderful things happen for love. Love heals. Love manages to build bridges from the old normal through no-man's land to the new normal. Even so, I advise my patients and their families and friends to speak to experts in matters of the heart. Get a psychologist into the boat for this trip. For what happens now is not a picturesque little joyride in a rowboat, but there is a rough sea, meter-high waves, utter disorientation in the spindrift and hungry fish everywhere. We have not learned any rules for this, or else we just started to compile our checklist. Do you remember?

People who have learned to regularly understand and solve problems will be able to transform the imminent crisis in a realistic manner – which can be relativized and managed. How well this succeeds, however, depends on how a person has lived until this moment. We are all the result of our past. Mature personalities are more crisis-proof.

People with their feet firmly in life can activate additional strength more easily. Nothing derails them just like that. Most importantly, they have freedom of choice. You are not born with it; you acquire it over the course of time, even though you may not have had the luck to grow up with an abundance of basic trust. In the end, it is about creating a sort of protected space inside oneself to which only people, animals and things are admitted that are good for us...and of course our beautiful memories, interests, and everything we are connected with in a special way. What gives us strength provides an anchor in our lives. The closer we are connected with things that are important to us, and the safer we feel in our inner protected space, the better we can overcome crises. Without a safe base, the amygdala will take command: fight or flight.

Do you know your inner protected space, this area within your soul? Has it changed over the years? And are the same people still by your side?

Times of crisis are crucial tests for friendships. Even though friendships are experienced more intensely than family relationships, they are terminable. Occasionally, a friend's nerves may be too weak for a hospital visit. It is usually impossible to repair such abandonment. When trust has suffered a crack, even the heart surgeon will give up; I have no suitable thread for such a wound. Yet I know that new people will suddenly appear on the horizon, as if they fell from the sky. Sometimes friends for life will first meet as fellow sufferers in hospital. I don't want to be annoying, but I have heard this comment, too: "Imagine, doctor, without the whole rubbish here I would never have met Ms. Baumann, and what would I have missed!"

10

IN THE VACUUM

Waiting.
    Waiting. Waiting.
      Waiting. Waiting. Waiting. Waiting. Waiting.
Waiting.
    Do something nice.
    Now, when it's still possible.
    Who knows how you'll fare after the clinic?
    You can put it behind you soon.
    I'm sure you'll manage.
    Oh, if only it were over already.
    Waiting.
    Now I would have time for all the things I like to do.
I could read or put together my model railroad, I could go for a
walk, sort my photos.
    But I can't.
    Waiting.
    How slowly a day passes.

I hope they don't postpone the date.

Everything annoys me.

I have to pull myself together, I'm spreading my bad mood.

What should I tell the boss when he asks when I'll come back – I just don't know?

My wife wants to have sex, but I can't. My head is so full. Even though there's nothing to do. Just waiting.

Waiting. Waiting. Waiting. Waiting. Waiting. Waiting. Waiting.

Supposing these are the last nice moments of my life. Supposing something goes wrong. Then I will be mad at myself for having spent my last days waiting, instead of doing nice things... while I still could.

Maybe I should cancel the operation?

I'm fed up with telling people on the phone that it's not time yet.

COVID is getting me down. I must not catch that now, no way. No one in my family can. Otherwise, they may not operate. Or there won't be a bed for me, as they are all taken by COVID patients. And what if my family isn't going to be allowed to visit me after the operation, and during rehab...if during the hardest time in my life I will lie utterly alone in an alien environment, cut off, isolated, desperate...

Yes, that could be the case. In the clinic where I work, many interventions were postponed. The patients who would have liked to delay the operation as long as possible, now realized how dearly they were longing for it: to live again unburdened, without this sword of Damocles hanging over their head. In my experience, the time interval between diagnosis and operation which is considered tolerable is different for each patient. Too fast, and they will have too little time to come to terms with the situation. Too slow, and they can become psychologically unstable. Occasionally, I will thus have a nervous wreck before me, and that is counterproductive as patients need their full strength for the operation and the time afterwards. COVID weighed many patients down with additional fears that they would get sick with the virus. The pandemic fills the intensive care wards. We need a bed in ICU with a ventilator after each of our operations. At least a heart can in many cases wait patiently for a few weeks even in an emergency, while other illnesses can end fatally during the waiting time: a cancer will not stop growing because the world happens to be in a pandemic. The waiting time is hard for the relatives, too, as they may have no strength left to comfort their loved ones again and again, to motivate them... always the same conversations, everything going round in circles.

In my opinion we must take action urgently: increase capacities, improve work processes, explore new options, so that the waiting times become shorter. Waiting too long makes you sick. Those who are familiar with relaxation techniques like yoga or breathing exercises are at an advantage, as people who have learned to meditate would know. Through meditation we learn to calm our thoughts. We breathe more deeply, which is good for the whole body. Ideally, meditation will give us composure and confidence. Fears will diminish. We learn to appreciate the moment and become more receptive to our sensory perceptions. Calmness allows us to draw new strength deep within us, and studies have revealed that meditation can ease pain.

There are many more good reasons to meditate, as one

thing is indisputable: our carousel of thoughts wears us out.

Have I done everything right in life?
　　I would have liked to still...
　　I would like to still...
　　I should have thought about this earlier.
　　What if it's over now.
　　That simply can't be.
　　I have planned so much still.
　　And my children.
　　My wife, my husband.
　　How quickly time has passed.
　　Should I have noticed something earlier?
　　Why does it happen to me of all people?
　　I would so much like to live as if everything were
fine.
　　To dance wildly once more.
　　Waiting.
　　And if something happens now?
　　I could have another stroke, what then?
　　The doctor said everything's still okay, that the aneurysm will not tear, but they are not looking inside me every day. What if he's wrong?

The patients have lost trust in their body. It let them down once already, did something it should not have done, bulged an artery or formed a tumor. How can you know it won't happen again? Some listen constantly to their inner voice. They no longer know what they're allowed to do and sometimes become utterly passive for fear of overstraining themselves. Or they constantly push themselves to their limits or beyond, believing this might be their last opportunity to enjoy life one more time. Then the relatives suffer and become sick with worry.

In many cases, I advise patients to live like before the diagnosis, provided their blood pressure is okay. "And if so far you've done ten kilometers on your bike on the weekend, do seven now."

In this way, patients can become used to a new normal in advance. I don't want to tell them that they will never do ten kilometers on their bike again, but they should not assume that after a heart operation everything would get back to what it was before. Those who insist on it make life hard for themselves.

Nights are the worst when everything is still, asleep. When you listen to the quiet breathing of the healthy person next to you. When your own heartbeat becomes so loud, fills the whole room. The world is divided into the healthy and the sick. A trench seems to separate them and over time becomes wider and wider. Waiting is not healthy, not good for the patients; we absolutely must shorten this time.

When I was still working in a transplantation team, I saw patients break down when they did not end up getting their "promised" heart. Patients who are waiting for a new heart sit next to their phone day and night, hoping for the crucial call. As soon as a suitable heart has been found, the clock is ticking on a time window of about four hours. Two teams work simultaneously, one traveling to the donor heart, the other preparing the patient for the operation. Yet sometimes something unexpected happens, and the patient is told: "We are sorry, the heart is not coming after all."

The longing for the old normal can become overpowering. We know our way around the normal, moving smoothly through our communities, families, and groups we belong to. But what happens to us now makes us an outcast. We no longer belong. We have something our normal companions don't have. Sure, there are groups in which everyone has it, but we don't yet know them – and do not want to get to know them, to be honest. Inwardly we feel like we belong to "the normal ones" – not to the self-help group for an illness, to people sharing a medical experience, or to any other marginal group. We want to get "back in", to belong.

Sometimes patients tell me that they long to go shopping or to drive their car from A to B, something very normal – and that they will forever enjoy it should they be able to do it again.

"Do you think it will end well?"

"We will do our best", I answer in such cases.

In this phase some patients will also ponder their death explicitly. They take stock, make their will, some plan their funeral. Others avoid such thoughts – for wouldn't they be a bad omen? The same is true for the relatives. Some push to hear the patient's last wishes, others do not want to know. Sometimes it will be helpful for the patient to speak with a friend or acquaintance who is not part of the inner family circle, who has an outside view, so to speak, and is more resilient. However, a layperson cannot replace a psychologist. Doctors would prefer to see the patient's advance directive to know how they would want us to act in an emergency.

Pretrial Confinement

Sometimes when I walk along our clinic's corridor and look into patients' faces, some of them remind me of the faces of defendants in movies. They are in "pretrial confinement", now sitting in front of a door behind which their trial will take place. They are called in, then the judgment will sound: "The defendant is found guilty of multiple counts of vessel calcification. The sentence is: five bypasses, to be carried out immediately."

The patients have visited the clinic a few times already, had appointments for preliminary examinations and conversations. But they went home the same day, except if their diagnosis required an overnight stay. This time around, they come in and don't go home. Will they ever be out in the fresh air again, will they leave the clinic on their own two feet or in a wheelchair or... be carried out in a box.

A rare but awful complication after vascular surgery is paraplegia. I will never forget the patient who after waking up reported with remarkable composure: "I can't move my legs anymore. Nevertheless, I'm infinitely grateful, because without the operation I wouldn't even know that I can't move my legs. I simply wouldn't be here, talking to you. Or else I'm dead and just don't know it, doctor?"

He looked at me as if he were in heaven, and in a way, he was: he had survived.

I visited this patient often, and most times his wife and daughter were sitting beside his bed. The three of them were planning his new life in a wheelchair. No one had expected anything like this, and yet they did not moan but instead quickly came to terms with a new normal. That really touched me – after all, this patient had been walking on his own two feet before the operation. His wife told me, a smile on her face: "We have to start from scratch again, think everything through again. The wheelchair will always remind us how lucky my husband was. I think our life will become even more precious now."

I am sure that this family had already been appreciative of life before. Studies prove that serious misfortunes do not necessarily make people depressive. Rather, they will – after some time, when they have processed what has happened to them – take up their quality of life at its former level. Those who go through life with ease will continue to do so even when they sit in a wheelchair. The same is true for grumblers. Both have gone through the same experience, but they live in different worlds. A remarkable finding of happiness research in this regard is that neither wealth nor beauty nor – and this perhaps is the most astonishing aspect – physical health correlate with a high level of happiness. The reverse conclusion is that a disappointment, loss, or serious misfortune do not exclude happiness and contentment. That provides us with something concrete to work with. And it makes the stay in pretrial confinement easier, too, as the divide which had existed in the family before – me sick, you healthy – now becomes visible. One remains in hospital, the other goes home – to a normal which has already stopped being one, as it is not normal for the one at home to sleep alone, in the same way as the hospital bed is not normal for the sick person. The latter is on the homestretch as they believe the operation is their goal. But it is only a stage. It does not matter how many times you remind patients of this; they do not want to hear it. For them, the operation is the finish.

Then it is time. Everything "on the outside" has been taken care of. Now the patient only has to hold out for two or three more days. Time changes. In a way, there is no time anymore. It has stopped, but then suddenly it speeds up. The patients think back over the recent past, or they look back deep into their life's history. Sometimes they recall an old holiday destination: I want to go back there one more time...if everything goes well. If everything goes well. That is often what they think while they say: it should be okay.

Has to.
> *Bad weeds grow tall.*
> *Here goes nothing.*
> *Don't worry.*
> *I'll pull through.*

In pretrial confinement patients can't act at their own discretion. They must follow the rules, they are woken up at a certain time, have their temperature taken and endure other strange things...and the food doesn't taste nice. So what if these were their last few meals?

"Last meal", he tried to joke with his wife.

"Don't say that", she retorted.

Nowadays patients no longer stroll through a clinic in their pajamas like in former times. Today they are dressed casually in tracksuits. Yet when someone never wears a tracksuit, it will constantly remind them of their situation now. I'm just imagining a patient's room with men in white shirts and ties, a suit jacket over their shoulders, and women in evening dresses. What an idea!

Patients can't leave the clinic. They feel incapacitated. If they have an appointment, they can't just go by themselves but are collected and escorted. They can't actively shape their life, it is taken from their hands. Occasionally a second diagnosis is added to the first one they already know. Big agitation! And suddenly the day is over. Where has it gone?

There follows another night when the ghosts crawl through the cracks. Will you see your son again? Will your family get by without you? Will there be enough money? And what if the operation as such goes well, but afterwards you won't function properly anymore? How long can love stand that?

One hears stories, so many stories. Some are of patients who weren't operated on despite their appointment because an emergency had to be brought forward. Sometimes they wish they were one themselves, so they could put it behind them. One hears so much. The day is long. The family comes in the afternoon.

"Soon it will be behind you."

It?

What, it?
The operation?
Or my whole life?

Disoriented. Lost. Lonely.
"Do you need something else for the night, Mr. Meier?", the nice nurse with the freckles asks.
"No thanks, it's all okay."
How often one says: it's all okay. When nothing's been okay for quite a while.
Nothing is valid anymore. But it's not the fault of the staff.
They are doing their best, even though they are really overworked.
You only notice when you're affected yourself what "nursing shortage" means.

Good Spirits

If things had gone according to plan, the nurse with the freckles would have gone home two hours ago. But nothing goes according to plan anymore. At least not according to plans made by people in high places who don't even know who will execute them at the bottom of the ladder, at a low wage.

One of them is the nurse with the freckles who, according to her friends, is much too good for the world. "You have to set limits", the family says. "Think of yourself for a change." But how could she when day after day she sees the shortages everywhere. "You've got helper syndrome!" She's heard that already, too, and thought to herself: thank God there are people like me, otherwise I would not know how we could care for the patients. But it is no longer pleasant. Nearly everything which attracted this nurse to her profession – and she has been working in it for quite some time – is gone. There is a lack of time particularly, and there are too few staff in the ward to manage the work. How are they supposed to find the time to do what the patients so urgently need: to hold a hand, to listen, to say a few nice words, and yes, to stay longer when things get tough, maybe even to the end. After all, who wants to die alone? And no one realizes, until one notices, oh my, we won't have to change the drip here anymore.

The nurse with the freckles says that today she would choose a different profession, and that she is sorry about it, but she has the impression at times that she is looking after documentation and machines more than people. I'm not nursing sick people but computers, is a thought she has had.

Oh whatever, I will stay with Mr. Meier for a few more minutes. She meant to look in on him her whole shift, but there simply wasn't time. Tomorrow he will have his big operation, unless it is called off again at the last minute like last time. That was horrible. Best not to think of it, not to let it get to me so much; it is better that way as there is nothing I can do. Otherwise, my conscience will be even worse, thinking that I'm not taking care of him properly – and then I won't get a wink of sleep again, as if it was *my* operation tomorrow. And I will have to be fit when there are only four of us in the ward.

Yes, nurses must be vigilant. They are the first staff members who the patients see in the clinic when they are admitted, and the last when they are discharged. Their assessment is important, too: how is the patient, what do we need to know, what should we watch out for, how stable are they at the moment, including psychologically? How can they find all this out when mostly they are busy using a computer, filling in forms? Nurses are so important, yet they are frequently neglected. They don't have the same lobbying power as doctors, they don't attend congresses, they are still not really appreciated by society – COVID has not changed much of that. They carry a whole clinic on their backs, and the wage is meager. I have seen countless nurses burn out, or else they become sluggish. Their daily stress has made them lose empathy, the very character trait which distinguished them and helps patients through hard times. A nice word, a heartfelt touch, a little joke, a caring question. The feeling to work for the patients, not against them. To see the patients as human beings, not as objects on which the service provider called nurse exercises their job. Consolation is a good word for what I mean: I am not alone, there is someone there who looks after me, even feels for me a little bit...

Patients usually feel closer to the nursing staff than to the doctors, who come and go and are somewhere high above. The nurses, on the other hand, who help with eating and washing and on the toilet, they are the good spirits. When there is time, they have lot of close contact with the patients, intensive moments, too; when they are pressed for time, however, they may perceive the patients as a burden: what does he want yet again, what is the matter this time. That is terrible, for both sides. The staff go home with the bad feeling of not having done enough, and the patients lie in their bed alone and forgotten and may not dare to ring for help even though everything hurts... but they do not want to be a nuisance and ask for the bed linen to be changed. Instead, they just lie there with their pain, and a small matter may become a big one.

This can have a variety of reasons. One is COVID-19. The fear of infection puts an extra strain on patients. Get vaccinated, to be sure? But will the vaccine be effective? And what if it does not agree with me? One of the most frequent questions from patients I had to answer in 2020 and 2021 was: "What happens if I get COVID, will you still operate?"

I answer them: "Your concern is legitimate. If your condition allows it, we would prefer to wait. If not, we will take additional protective measures like for patients with AIDS or hepatitis."

Fear will not grip every person, but many. No two fears are the same, and fear can manifest itself very differently. What is certain is that it is hard for most people to say: "I'm afraid." Silence, on the other hand, can make them very lonely, even more so when they want to keep up their old roles at all costs. But there is an entry point for a conversation at every key step of the graph (see above at the end of the chapter OPENING). Our foundation aims to make these entry points visible, and to show how we can meet every patient exactly where they are to provide company, comfort, and personalized measures.

Role Plays

Now is also a good time to say goodbye to our roles. Roles are useful in everyday life; they often help us as we know automatically how to behave. But there is a difference between doing things automatically and living. We all "play" different roles in our life. We are children and parents, bosses and employees, the clown in the sports club and the worrywart in the neighborhood. For every person we meet we take on different roles, even if they are only marginally different. When two old friends meet, their wives may later say: that wasn't at all like you.

Yes, you slide into your old role, it gives you the feeling of safety. You return to the place, to the behavior you once learned. But when roles solidify, become set in stone, we forfeit our liveliness. If for example we cling to the role of "strong man" or "brave woman" even though we feel entirely different at the moment, this would be a good time to ask what would happen if we were to question or even abandon this role. After some irritation, the whole playing field would change – which could be good for everyone involved.

But it can also create fear, which is why psychological support is sensible here. It is possible, however, to do a quick assessment of your roles. Do I still like them? Do they still fit me? Which would I like to suspend for a while? One does not have to shed them forever but can simply experiment a little, slide into another one; the fund is inexhaustible. We could also act super brave for a change – and be without any role whatsoever. Yes, when are we ever like that? Who am I when I'm my "naked self"? This anxious patient? Or is that also only a role, and we are all acting in a play set in a hospital – and now the heart surgeon makes their entrance?

To be fully alive means to recognize change. We are all constantly changing. We don't have to always be the same. We are allowed to try out things in life. And when something did not go so well in the past, one reason may be that we were in the wrong role at the wrong moment; it may suit at another time.

A woman asked me to talk to her husband. "He is beside himself because they put him in a room facing north."

The patient's north was called fear, which was so big that I could see his heartbeat through his shirt. He had a pulse of 140 during our whole conversation. But fear? Him? No, definitely not. It was just that this room did not agree with him.

"My husband is not afraid of anything", his wife confirmed. She desperately wanted to believe this, because if her husband was afraid of something, she would have to be afraid herself.

While I had a chat alone with him, the patient's pulse slowed down.

"What on earth did you say to my husband?", the wife enquired curiously.

"I'm sorry, that comes under medical confidentiality."

"But my husband and I have no secrets."

"In which case he will surely tell you everything."

"You could do that, too."

"As I said, confidentiality."

"Would that also apply if I were to tell you something?"

"Absolutely."

"But I am not your patient."

"It applies."

"Well, there is something weighing on his heart…"

Religious people find comfort and hope from their God during times of hardship and crises, which often helps them master these times more easily. They draw strength from their prayers. Thus, there is always a course of action for them, they are not powerless and can turn to their God. This allows them hope and gives them composure: whatever happens, they cannot fall deeper than into God's hands. Those who only fall into the hands of the demigods in white may land hard. Which I want to avoid at all costs.

In our clinic, we are collecting data from which we can conclude how to best help our patients. I would like to see us identify types and groups which we then assign to each patient, so that they can get the best possible preventative treatment. This would save serious money for our health system, as we do not react only when something is going in the wrong direction but ensure from the start that things are on a good path, specifically for this patient.

I have been supporting patients through the process for many years now, and I know that they handle it all better and are less prone to postoperative complications when they realize exactly what happens and when. That they are not alone and lost but that what is happening now is normal, even though they do not yet know this normal and never wanted to know it. Nevertheless, it is the normal transition from one life to another.

In your old life you may have done lots of exercise and were proud of your time in the one-thousand-meter race. In your new life you will run a little more slowly. That is okay. Be happy that you're still able to run. Don't force yourself to perform and overstrain yourself because your situation has changed. Life is beautiful nevertheless, or now more so than ever. Change disciplines: a four-hundred-meter race is a physical challenge, too. It is just that new limits are in place. If you move within these limits, your quality of life will increase. If, on the other hand, you only strive to transgress these limits, things will be arduous for you. Do you want that? Sure, you can decide to use all your energy to get everything back to what it was. But it may be that you would only be playing a role – that of who you were before. But you are no longer that person.

What is so bad about that?

Maybe it is quite nice?

Could you allow that?

Things may also turn out differently, by the way. A woman recovered so well after her operation that she was positively bursting with energy. Her husband, who had become used to the cozy life at the side of a heart patient, found it hard to keep up and confided in me: "Well, I found it more comfortable before."

Every now and then I meet patients who enjoy being the focus of attention when they are sick. There are even those who like to stay in the clinic as long as possible. Are these always the lonely ones? Whom no one is waiting for at home? I don't think so. Once a successful woman, mother of two children, who lived in a happy marriage, told me: "My illness taught me how nice it is when someone looks after you. When I was sick as a child, my mother would look after me but sort of like a service provider. The special treatment I needed was annoying to her. Here I enjoyed so much heartfelt attention and care by my family and also in the hospital. I was able to relax completely. That was a very important experience for me. I was able to make up for a small part of my childhood, and I am very grateful for it."

"But that's enough now", interjected her husband who was present during the conversation. "It's not that now you will have to be constantly sick." He turned to me: "That happens, doesn't it? People who like to be patients because that makes them the center of attention?"

"Yes", I replied. "But that isn't my area of expertise."

"But you are the heart specialist!", the man joked.

"*You* are the specialist for your wife's heart, and I think…" I winked at them both. "You're managing quite well."

Thus, it turns out that the vacuum is far from empty. There is a lot in there, and it goes very, very deep. It is my desire to offer individual help for patients to manage it, so that they may better find their way and know they are not alone. Not even during the night before the big event.

The Night Before

I am convinced, and studies confirm it, that a confident patient who feels safe and secure has better chances of a positive outcome. I usually visit my patients once more in their ward on the evening before the operation, even though the preoperative conversation has long happened. Because I know: this night is the worst, the essence of the past weeks and months. Fear of death. Agonizing questions. Will I be able to teach my son how to swim? If, if, if. Will I see my parents again? How will my wife cope without me?

Do we doctors realize this? We are human beings, too, and who wants to confront someone else's fears, let them get close…no thank you. I am here as a surgeon, not as a psychologist or…a human being? But what will happen to me if I switch off my being human? Sure, in the operating room I will work with utmost professionalism. But now…when I sit by the bed of the patient, me who tomorrow morning will do the unfathomable and cut them open, and advance to regions untouched by anyone else that even the patients themselves can't see. Deep, deep inside them. I will not only touch their heart but shut it down or take it out of the thorax. I might connect their circulation to a heart-lung machine, work inside their thorax with different metal instruments such as retractors, forceps, and suture clips.

Every patient is different, every conversation goes differently even when the same questions are asked. I stay until I sense that the patient is calmer. Tonight, I do not want them to be desperate but optimistic. I would like them to inwardly agree, to trust me, for them to decide of their own accord to place their heart not in any surgeon's hands but in *mine*. For me, that is not just a nice gesture but an indispensable necessity. Self-determined, the patient should shake the hand which will touch him so deeply. We are now a team and look after their heart together.

"It will be okay, doctor, won't it?"

"I will give my best, and you will give your best."

Later I often hear after you visited me I was even able to sleep.

One day, a patient from abroad came to our clinic for

an operation. It was his third heart surgery, and he had made arrangements in case he should not survive it. This included having asked his brother to wait for the outcome of the operation in the clinic with his wife, so she would not be alone should there be news of his death. He told me all this the night before the operation. His wife did not know any of this, but told me the day after the successful operation that her husband had mentioned my visit to her and how it had changed his mood to being positive. That had calmed her down as well, especially since the nights before his two previous operations had been so bad for her as if she herself had been the one to undergo the operation. No, she corrected, even worse.

And I? I often fall asleep with the thought of tomorrow's patient. Then sometimes something unforeseen will happen, an emergency; I get up at 3am and drive to the clinic in a hurry. And later I will again stand next to the bed of the patient whose operation has been postponed. One day, though, he will lie before me, and as I have come to know him, he is more to me than a surgical area covered with sterile drapes. I have talked to him, he told me of his granddaughter, and now I am looking deeply into him. Yes, it is harder, but also easier, at least for me. For this is why I became a doctor: to heal human beings, not just sections of them. What may sound like an expenditure of time isn't one in reality. Sometimes it takes only two or three minutes; to establish intensity is not a matter of time, but of the willingness of two human beings to connect. We all know this: some encounters with others were very short, and yet they changed our life or created a lasting memory. As medical professionals, we can shape the encounters with our patients. We will experience that the good that we do will come back to us.

Many studies examine the question of what really helps patients. Our patient has now fallen asleep, and I will use the time of his last night before the operation to give you a little insight into different possibilities of disease management. Then we will wake up the patient and begin.

Disease Management

In a crisis, every person displays individual reactions based on their experiences and prehistory. By getting to know them as thoroughly as possible, we can offer them tailor-made disease management. In this way we can act purposefully to absorb the existing or expected strain psychologically, emotionally, and mentally. How easy it is to say: you have to learn to accept your illness. But that is far from easy, and many patients feel pressured by such requests. They may even put pressure on themselves if they enter the process of dealing with their illness with very high expectations.

Another approach in medicine and psychology concentrates on quality of life rather than acceptance, even if the latter is part of it and enters through the backdoor, so to speak. In this approach, we primarily ask how patients perceive their illness with all its implications and side effects; that is also the aim of the matter closest to my heart I mentioned above (see towards the end of the chapter OPENING). We ask which changes the illness will cause in patients' normal life, always with the quality of life in focus. To find answers, we must turn to the patients as human beings, because quality of life is a subjective condition. The patients will immediately feel they are being seen differently. Even just our enquiring about their quality-of-life signals to them: we are not merely interested in getting you back on your feet as quickly as possible so you function again, contribute to the gross national product and do not lead to unnecessary costs. Rather, we want you to be well and your quality of life to be the best possible.

This stress-free approach relaxes the patients. They can let go. They don't have to – they are allowed to. They may have made plans previously about how soon they want to make progress. Now they will ask, maybe for the first time, about what they want, what is good for them. They ponder what their quality of life might look like once they have put everything behind them. So, they don't ask: will I function again? But rather: will I be able to enjoy things, feel joy, be together happily with others? That is a totally different approach, one in which the patients naturally participate more willingly. The concept is summed up in the term "compliance": the patients' willingness to accept the proposed therapy and support it through their own cooperation, which will increase enormously if the aim of the therapy is good quality of life. In that case, I as a patient will be firmly and zealously committed to the therapy – much more than if the goal was to merely put me back together.

This kind of care can also tear down some walls between doctors and patients, as they now share a common goal: quality of life. Mind you, the goal has merely been renamed, but before there was danger that doctors would force measures onto patients which would hamper their quality of life. One example: everyone knows that smoking is harmful, but when a patient of mine wants to smoke a cigarette while drinking a cup of coffee in the afternoon, and when that represents a good quality of life for them, I will not put him off their cigarette by mentioning the commonplace that smoking is not healthy.

The same goes for a glass of wine in the evening. My hope is that my patient wants to enjoy this life as long as possible and will therefore voluntarily ditch the cigarette and not have a second glass of wine.

So much for the theory. In practice, we distinguish four styles of coping with a crisis. In most cases, people lean towards one of them. However, to find the one most suitable for them, they can try them all; a preference will quickly emerge. As the saying goes: the leopard can't change its spots.

It is important not to explain to a patient who has identified with a style of coping that it is the wrong approach. If an illness denier and a meaning seeker clash, they will not benefit from each other and inspire each other as long as one tries to convince the other that they are wrong. The illness denier may call the meaning seeker a wimp, and the meaning seeker may take the illness denier as a person who shirks the conscious examination of him/herself. The tricky part is noticing which pattern a patient or person-in-crisis prefers, and then to act within this framework when one wants to make a meaningful contribution. We learn that elsewhere in life, too: it is pointless to want to transfer one's own convictions to others. If we do that, failure is inevitable. It is better to meet people where they are. And that is what we will do now.

1. **Denial**

One wants to have as little as possible to do with what has happened. Critics will say: "You are putting your head in the sand." But one just does not want to deal with it, because it's pointless anyway. On top of that, one does not have time for laments and little ailments. Critics will say: "If only you had looked after yourself better, if only you weren't..."

"That's none of your business", the denier will say and won't want to talk about it anymore. His view of the world is not wrong. It is a positive thing not to make a crisis bigger than it is. A patient with a coping style of denial approaches a crisis as normally as possible. No dramas please. Someone like that won't let things get them down.

This attitude reduces feelings of helplessness and being at someone's mercy which many sick people suffer from. Thus, it increases the quality of life. By and large, it is a good strategy, if you don't suppress what happened completely. To prevent that, helpful suggestions to correct one's course may be appropriate.

2. Seeking Meaning

What is the meaning of my illness? Why me, of all people? What is the hidden message? Where did my life take a wrong turn? What should I learn from this illness?

As humans we are inclined to explain the world to ourselves and look for connections whenever there is something we do not understand. Conspiracy theories feed off this need. Thus, meaning seekers hunt for the hidden meaning in the crisis, for an inner logic. We find it easier to accept events when we fabricate a story which explains why things got to where they are.

The weak point: One may lapse into brooding and can slide further into a depression. That, however, is something we absolutely do not need at this point.

Another "course correction" might be suggested here, as otherwise the dangerous question of guilt may arise. Most of the time, there is an obvious guilty party in car crashes or crimes of fraud; in any case, it is a matter for a court of law. In contrast, the guilt for an illness can only rarely be identified, and patients will often sit in judgment on themselves: "Why me? How did I become guilty? Or is it not me but my financial worries, my genes, my work colleagues, or the cellphone poles?"

Those who believe in astrology may hold a star constellation responsible for their fate. Someone else acknowledges that for years they have been in the wrong marriage. Yet another believes for the illness to be a hint to change their life fundamentally. Great – if better quality of life is the result. In general, one should try not to get caught up in the carousel of thoughts which asks about meaning, as asking why does not lead to better quality of life. It would be better to ask: "And now…what will I make of this?" Those who follow the next strategy will have good answers.

3. Attack

The illness or crisis is a challenge and is accepted as such. Even more – it will be classified from the start as conquerable, as one won't be acquiescent. Such people do not only go through all the available therapies and suggestions, but they also actively look for information and alternatives and immerse themselves in the problem. Self-help groups are havens for those who thrive on an active style of coping. All this gives them a good feeling of being on top of the situation. They want to control their illness and its implications rather than being dominated by them.

4. **Support**

Support is also a form of activity, but in this case, it is mostly about sharing the burden of the illness with family, friends and other people. Those with a high social competence can utilize it in a crisis.

As I mentioned at the start, as social beings we need other humans. We want to belong, to speak openly, to get and give advice, to be needed – and all this we only experience in an encounter with other people. This is of special importance during an illness, and those who embrace such encounters will find much strength through the support of others. The closeness of kind people changes the chemical processes in the brain and reduces stress hormones. To have friends protects you from stress and lets you heal faster after illnesses, as positive social relationships coincide with the distribution of brain chemicals such as oxytocin, endorphins, and dopamine, which convey happiness and fend off the physical effects of stress.

However, one would have to have built this support previously, and one must not overuse it. When one constantly displays signs of helplessness, one becomes a burden for others and creates difficulties for them. Relatives usually want to help someone who needs support, but if their readiness to help is overused, conflicting emotions accrue which can heavily afflict them. How can I feel so adversarial when someone needs help! The help is given nevertheless, but rather as a duty, which may strain the relationship further.

An over-display of independence is also not a good way to secure support. Those who constantly point out that they can manage by themselves will affront people who would give support with all their heart but are not allowed to.

A good compromise would be to make it clear that the strain is extremely high at the moment, but that the sufferer takes responsibility and will accept support on this basis. Support is different from demanding that the others carry one through life on their shoulders, so to speak. It becomes even more irksome if this is not demanded but quietly expected. And when it is not given, the sick will sulk…and there may be ill feelings during an illness. Open communication is better, as all things unspoken will impede the process of coping.

We are not always the same person in our day-to-day life, and the same applies for the way in which we deal with an illness. There are good days and there are bad days. It depends on many factors. Pain comes in spurts. The weather can play a role, as can the side effects of the medication and our social environment. A person can utilize all of the coping styles, but at any given time there will be a preference. Usually, we do not notice which course we follow. By becoming aware of it and realizing that there are further possibilities, we may correct our course here and there. It is a matter of the heart for me to support the approach of my patients, and I want to motivate my colleagues, too, to support the impulse which comes from the patients themselves.

We have determined in our past how we will deal with a severe illness, a crisis, our fate – and we determine our future today. How well someone can manage and eventually overcome an illness, depends on different psychosocial influences, including our childhood. This is why personal conversations are so important, because as doctors we can find out the extent of the hardship if we listen closely. There are different ways to measure this, for example standardized questionnaires which determine the psychosocial strain for chronic illnesses. One falls ill, accepts the illness and is one's old self again. Many painful processes and changes come along with this. We must never forget how much the patients' self-confidence, self-perception and self-efficacy suffer.

It is scientifically proven that how one deals with an illness will affect the course of the illness and the quality of life. If coping with the crisis is not successful, professional help should be sought. After all, we have been through so much already, so now it is time to choose a shortcut. This is a meaningful way for us to learn to deal with the illness and integrate it in our life. Then we will live with it rather than against it. That is a fight we cannot win in any case.

Depending on how used to engaging with their psychological constitution a person is, they will turn inward after an operation or illness. We often say: "It took a long time for me to realize this" or "It took time before I came to terms with it." The healing of the body can occur faster than the healing of the soul. Of course, not everyone who is severely ill is in a bad mood. On the other hand, everyone who encounters a person in dire straits can make a difference. As human beings we are constantly interacting with our environment. Outside influences like stress do not only change our immediate condition but can prevent the activation of certain gene segments in the long run. That impacts not only ourselves, but our environment, too, through the change in our behavior. An illness never hits only the body; it is always the whole human being that is affected, including their soul.

But now let us go back to our patient whom we visited last night...do you remember?

11

THE INTERVENTION

Usually, patients don't sleep so well before the operation, not even if we had a chat the previous evening. I, too, have a lot on my mind in the night before the operation, even though operations are part of my everyday normal. I go through the upcoming intervention one more time on the drive to the clinic. There are operations we call routine, while others are big and difficult. Yet even during one that has been classified as "easy", complications can occur at any moment. A bleeding can be impossible to stop, for example, or the heart won't start after the shutdown, or many other things. It is nevertheless very rare for a patient to die on the operating table. Most patients leave the OR alive, even though sometimes their life might be hanging by a thread. The next hours and days will show if the thread breaks.

I am not content with a Plan A during my preparation for the operation. I always have Plans B, C, D and E. I make myself aware of the procedures in each of these plans: if that happens, I will do this. After so many operations, these are partly routine matters for me, but it is very important to recall them time and time again.

The patient, too, will now have the operation on their mind – without thinking of complications, I hope. Ideally, they concentrate on Plan A: everything will be fine.

While I am in my car, on the way to the clinic, the patient in their bed will be wheeled to the waiting room, where they are identified for the second time; the first identification had happened before in their room. Every ward has its own checklist, which is ticked off meticulously. Later I will collect the patient from the waiting room and accompany them to the operating room. The patient is not alone in the waiting room; there are other patients waiting for their surgery or recovering after an emergency operation. It is not so rare that we operate in the middle of the night, as sometimes every minute counts – or even, for matters of the heart, every second.

A patient is agitated as they face the biggest adventure of their lives. Someone will reach into their body; people will look into their open thorax. They will do things there that the patients may well not want to imagine. And yet this is their only chance to continue to live. Their hope is big, infinitely big… and their fear, too.

Once I arrive at the hospital, there is a handover. The colleagues from the ICU nightshift inform the dayshift about the night's events. I think it is crucial to mention the patients by name. So, none of this: "the valve's ok, the bypass had a crisis, we had to reanimate the aortic rupture". How we speak, after all, is how we think; I don't want my patients reduced to building sites. I prefer it like this: "Everything is ok with Mrs. Müller after the heart valve procedure. Mr. Meier had a crisis during the night after his bypass operation. And we had to reanimate Mr. Schmied at around 3am; he is stable now." If I hear names, I see the whole human being, whom I know a little bit as I make sure I get an idea about all of my patients in ICU. In this way, I am literally "in the picture", even though the handover happens on the computer. About twenty colleagues are involved.

After the handover, I go to the surgical ward to collect my patient – his name is Richard Schwarz – from the waiting room. This "collection" became standard at our clinic in the Netherlands in 2020. I find this fantastic and would like to see it happen internationally, and the conversation the night before. A few kilometers away in Germany – where I also operate, in the town of Aachen – the procedures look very different. I deem the process in the Netherlands more humane, and thus more successful, for patients, nursing staff and doctors.

I spend eighty percent of my time operating in the Netherlands, and twenty percent in Germany. Even though the two clinics aren't even forty kilometers (25 miles) apart, the two health systems are fundamentally different, especially as euthanasia is permitted in the Netherlands and some patients decide against an operation in favor of a dignified death.

While in Germany we are used to only the boss having a say, they mostly forego hierarchies in the Netherlands. I find this way of working considerably more relaxed. I turned my back on the German system to a degree a few years ago, because it does not seem constructive to me when your number-one priorities are the patients' dignity and quality of life. Too often it is about case numbers. Surgeons have to crank out products, that is to say operations; they do not have time for their patients and are trained to be service providers – for customers or better still for insurance companies, and private ones if possible. With three operations scheduled in one day, there is no time to get to know a patient; it is reminiscent of a conveyor belt. While my assistant does the suturing, I already prepare for the next procedure, and enter operating room two where another assistant has already opened the thorax. I do my job, then move on to operating room three where another patient, thorax, lies open on a table. During my many years as a heart surgeon in Germany, I may have got to know about a third of my patients. Of the others, only their hearts. That went against my inner conviction, even though I also experienced many beautiful moments in the German clinics. The aim in Germany is to operate as much as possible; the numbers have to add up. They have to add up in the Netherlands, too, but a different path is used to get there.

I don't want to generalize. I can only talk about my experiences. I would like for Germany to look at its neighbors: what are they doing better? As a young man I wanted to study in Germany because the country had such a good reputation. "Made in Germany" was a seal of quality. That should not only apply to technology, though. How about a quality seal for being humane? The word for it exists already: kindhearted.

Another thing I like about the Netherlands is that the equality of men and women exists as a matter of course.

Female heart surgeons have it tough in Germany, whereas in the Netherlands the surgeon's gender does not matter, only their competence.

As I had sat beside Richard Schwarz's bed the night before, I can now take up our conversation when I greet him in the waiting room. Usually, patients are so tense and in their own world, in the long dark tunnel that represents their journey, that they are grateful for a little small talk. Often, I hold a patient's hand during the journey down the long corridor from the waiting area to the operating room. No words are required. I sense two things: besides the relief that we will start now, fear is the patient's dominating emotion. Most try not to let it show. Depending on the personality type, some say something funny, while others are very quiet and yet others once again express their trust in me: "Doctor, I rely on you."

"We will both give our best", I reply.

It is an indescribable situation, to go along this corridor hand in hand with this stranger who at this moment is so very close to me. We are connected by fate. Although he is operated on by a whole team, without whom I could never undertake this procedure, I am the ship's captain. I want to bring my passenger safely to the shore of his new life. At the same time, I also need to watch my crew.

That crew usually comprises my assistant doctor, a surgical nurse with their assistant (the so-called circulating nurse), the anesthetist with their assistant, the perfusionist responsible for the heart-lung machine, and their assistant. Our teams are mixed in all positions, so there are also female perfusionists, male nurses, female anesthetists etc. There is no linguistic distinction in

Dutch; for example, both male and female cardiologists are called "cardioloog".

Even if I feel a little nervous before a very difficult operation, my team is not to notice it. I am the captain. I am the one keeping track of things. If I give the impression of being insecure, everyone would be affected. The confidence with which I approach this task will spread to my team. I am balanced and controlled; I don't have to make a special effort as that is my mentality. I must mediate when there are any disagreements between members of my team. Like in many other professions, these teams are not assembled by request: rosters are created, and you sail with a different crew every day. It is in the nature of things, of humans specifically, that not everyone gets along with everyone else. To balance that is part of my job as a leader.

It is also important to me that the mood in the OR is good. Everyone knows we're not here to have a party, but sometimes music helps brighten the mood. I have different playlists for different operations. We share one goal: to see the patient safely to their new normal. I remind my team of that once more. We will all give our best, exactly as we discussed. Before the operation, I tell the team about every single planned step and point out what we will do if something does not go as planned. Our teamwork will be strengthened by this safeguard of knowing that all critical moments have been considered. At the end of our checklist in the OR I remind my crew that we will have a debriefing during which everyone can explain how they fared. We can give and receive feedback. I am very aware that every team can only be as strong as its weakest member. During heart surgery, you must not be afraid of physical contact; we stand so close to each other at the table that I can see my assistant's every pore.

When we operate on premature infants, our hands are nearly bigger than the small human's body. Some weigh just over one pound. They are operated on under a heat lamp. A healthy infant's blood vessel, which in the womb went from the heart past the lungs, will close of its own accord within hours or days after birth. However, that often does not happen with premature infants, and when all other measures fail, we have to operate to close the so-called ductus, as it misdirects the blood which circles between heart and lung rather than going to the organs like it should. During such an operation, we nearly stand on each other's toes. A surgical nurse once told me that she is sometimes overcome by the desire to pop pimples when we're in the thick of the procedure.

Most people have no idea how physically demanding a surgeon's profession is. You are bent forward slightly when you work, sometimes for seven or eight hours without eating, drinking, or going to the toilet. We get so close to each other, as if we were members of the same family; we smell each other's shower gels, but hopefully not perfume or sweat. You learn to defer your needs. In the OR, blood and other fluids are only for the patients.

Crew Only

Not all of the colleagues I mentioned work in the sterile area at the table. In the OR we distinguish between the sterile area and the nonsterile area. The surgical nurse, the assistant doctor and I are in the sterile area; all others are outside of it. The circulating nurse hands the instruments to us from the nonsterile to the sterile area. Each instrument has multiple layers of wrapping.

When the circulating nurse takes it from the nonsterile area, they remove one layer, hand it into the sterile area where the surgical nurse removes the second before it is used at the table. The magic circle between sterile and nonsterile is one meter wide. On no account must the patient come in contact with something nonsterile. That is why on TV one sometimes sees a nurse wipe the sweat from the surgeon's forehead. That is not a labor of love towards the surgeon, but towards the patient. Sweat in a wound is a high risk. Luckily, I do not sweat during an operation, difficult as it may be, not even under the heat lamp when I am operating on premature infants.

Germs are our great invisible enemy in the OR. They can cause horrific wound infections and much suffering for patients, who we will not be able to discharge after five or six days even though the operation went well. When a wound infection gets out of hand, that can result in a hospital stay of many weeks. The patient will be in the clinic for a long time, sometimes with an open thorax, because the wound won't heal. It is a long process full of setbacks to clean it so it will finally close; for the patient, that is a horrible ordeal.

As this is such a serious problem, hygiene is the clinic's alpha and omega. Correct and thorough disinfection also shows respect and appreciation for the patient. Ignaz Semmelweis, the pioneer of hospital hygiene, was laughed at and called crazy about one-hundred and fifty years ago because of his hygiene instructions, which many deemed exaggerated. If they had taken his findings seriously, many people would have been spared a lot of suffering. But back then it was not yet known that bacteria cause illnesses. It is tragic when a successful operation ends in disaster because of germs.

The topic of sterility is of such great importance that it lingers after the operation. After a long procedure, when I am at home cooking (which relaxes me), it may well happen that I ask my wife: "Is the frying pan sterile?", or that she reminds me that I am no longer in the OR when I forget the "please" when I ask for a knife.

While I am collecting my patient from the waiting room, my team prepares. The surgical nurse sets her table. Are all instruments there? The perfusionist checks the machine. Everything happens according to checklists. For the anesthetist as well. When I arrive in the OR with the patient, they all welcome him nicely. Every member of the team introduces themselves by name. "Good morning Mr. Schwarz, I am Dr. Daniele, your anesthetist." – "Good morning Mr. Schwarz, I am surgical nurse Karin." And so on. Depending on the patient's condition, a few more words may be exchanged. "It's really foggy this morning, but when you wake up, I'm sure it will be sunny."

The next step is hard, maybe the hardest for the patient – after all, he will sleep through what happens later. Now he must transfer from his bed onto the operating table. If he can't manage himself, he will get help. He is wearing nothing but his patient gown which is open at the back. He exposes himself to looks from strangers, which is a fragile moment for many patients. His bareness makes him terrifyingly aware of what is about to happen; it is a symbol of his utter helplessness. He is lying down while everyone else is standing over him. As soon as the patient is on the operating table, we cover him with a blanket. The patients are often cold. I may squeeze his cold hand one more time, or someone else will. We tell him: "Now our anesthetist will take care of you, you have already met her. As soon as you're deeply asleep, we will begin the operation like we discussed. When we're done, I will call your family like we said. I have the number ready."

I think it is important that the patient falls asleep with this information. Once more I squeeze his hand, then step away. The anesthetist identifies the patient yet again and asks if he is fasting, has any allergies, and some other things, just to be safe. During the next thirty to forty-five minutes, the anesthetist and their assistant will prepare the patient for the operation. First there will be a prick into his hand for an arterial catheter and an infusion. The patient will still feel this, but none of what happens from now on. The anesthetic is administered, and he falls asleep. He won't feel the breathing tube which will be placed in his windpipe, or the central venous catheter in his neck, or the urine catheter in his urethra. Finally, the patient is connected to all important measuring devices. The patient is cleared by the anesthetist, and he is sterilized by the surgical nurse who washes him with disinfectant. The patients in Aachen are orange, in Maastricht they are purple. Sterile drapes are fixed around the patient. Nearly time to begin. For me, too.

After copious handwashing, during which I go through the operation in my mind again step by step, I will be clad by the surgical nurse. She holds the gown up for me, I step into it, make a few turns in a sort of green-gown choreography, and finally slip into the gloves which are held out to me. When I step to the operating table, everyone has taken their position. Everything which is handed into the sterile area is double-wrapped and will now be unwrapped, including the tubes of the heart-lung machine which will come into contact with the patient.

Beating Hearts

With the scalpel I cut the skin, starting at the sternum. Only the skin. Then I take the electrical knife. It splits and at the same time separates fat tissue and musculature in a way that there is no bleeding. This is an unpleasant moment, as the burned flesh stinks. But our knife has a good suction device which quickly makes the smoke vanish. To be able to work on the patient's body using electricity, we need an arrester, grounding. For this reason, a plate has been attached to the patient, neutralizing electricity. He would suffer burns if we were to forget this.

For me as an operator, the electric knife can be painful, too – when my glove has a hole. This has happened three times so far, and each time I got an electric shock. Once even the tweezers, with which I had just lifted a little vessel, flew through the air. I told my assistant to put electricity on the vessel, as I did not know that my glove had a hole. Some surgeons always wear two pairs of gloves, not just nowadays with the high risk of infection by COVID. Generally, we all pay attention to our gloves and those of our colleagues – not only to protect ourselves but of course the patients as well.

The beep-beep-beep, the patient's pulse, will be with us for the next hours. We do not hear it consciously, and yet everyone is alarmed when it changes considerably or indeed falls silent. This may not signify anything bad, sometimes it is only that an electrode has come off. In that case, someone from the nonsterile area will crawl under the sterile green table and reattach it. For the whole duration of the intervention, the anesthetic team will monitor the patient's sleep. Anesthetics can be finely dosed nowadays. Observing the brain waves and other parameters, the colleagues can see at any time how deep the patient's anesthesia is.

The tension is palpable until we have connected the patient to the heart-lung machine and work with a safety net, so to speak. My assistant has been busy with the patient's legs for a while. That is why they are purple from the disinfectant, too, as we will take out the veins for the bypasses here. Their job will then be taken over by other vessels, which will become buddy vessels: all for one, and one for all. The body's vessels form a superb network. If the normal blood flow is blocked somewhere, smaller vessels called collaterals take over. However, that works only to a certain degree. If an important vessel in the heart area closes, the buddies cannot fulfil its part completely; decompensation occurs – a heart attack.

When we have sawn through the sternum and stopped the bleeding, we spread the ribs and look inside the thorax. Under it, there is the heart sac, where the heart lies. We use the versatility of this flexible and at the same time tear-resistant sac, called pericardium, when we have to repair a heart valve or stitch up a hole somewhere, for example one that is the consequence of an innate heart defect. We can already see the heart's movements well through the pericardium. Next, we create access to the "heart of the matter". Now it lies before us.

"Hello, heart!"

Sometimes I touch it – it is as if I would shake hands with it. In fact, I take it into my hand and examine its surface, where the coronary vessels can be seen: which size are they? After all, here is where we want to attach the bypasses.

The heart is not used to being touched. It does not like

it, starts to jolt and stumble. It is resisting. I let go of it, as we are not yet in the safe zone, connected to the heart-lung machine.

I am totally absorbed in everything I do. I have no thoughts. I identify myself with every movement of my hand, while at the same time I notice every noise: the beeping of the heartbeat, comments from the team. Now and then the human being before me flashes through my mind – what we talked about, what I know about him. It is hard to fathom that I am now looking deep inside him. This miracle fascinates me time and time again. The most compelling experience for me is when I have not only opened the thorax, but the abdomen as well – then I can freely look into the whole body. On the one hand, it seems like something forbidden, as a body is not made to be opened and "offer" itself like this. On the other hand, there is great allure, like x-ray with flesh and blood. I can look down to the spine, recognize the intestines and all organs, moved by the heartbeat which we are about to stop with a potassium solution. In preparation, we attach string sutures to the vessels and heart, in order to be able to insert the cannulas and tubes. As soon as the machine is connected, it takes over the functions of heart and lung. We see the heart become empty. Just then it filled and emptied with powerful pumping action; now it becomes limp. The heart stands still.

Communication in the team happens according to the checklist, question-and-answer style.

"Aorta is clamped", I say.

The perfusionist repeats: "Aorta is clamped."

In this way, I can be sure that the information has reached him.

I say to the anesthetist: "Blood pressure is too high."

She repeats: "Blood pressure is too high. I will give him something."

"Okay, you will give him something", I say.

My assistant has finished preparing the veins. We now begin to expose the coronary arteries and attach the bypasses. At the end, the heart is vented, and the aortic clamp removed. The blood which can flow from the heart-lung machine to the heart gradually flushes out the potassium solution. Then the bypasses which we sutured to the heart are connected to the aorta, so that the blood can take this new path. The old vessels are dysfunctional, and we won't touch them; the blockage will progress further – but now there is a detour. A bypass operation does not reverse calcification, it only serves as protection against a (further) heart attack. We check thoroughly if everything is tight, and hope that the heart will resume its work without complications when we disconnect it from the heart-lung machine. We have also begun to thicken the blood again, which we had thinned considerably so that no clots form when the patient is connected to the machine.

Everything is going according to plan. We temporarily attach a pacemaker to the myocardium; the pacemaker's lead comes out through the abdominal wall. Then we insert tubes to drain away the discharge from the wound. Finally, the sternum is clamped with steel wires – this is the sturdiest and cleanest solution. These wires will remain in the patient's body forever, unless they cause discomfort, which can sometimes happen. The bone will heal and grow back together within two to three months.

Usually, I leave the suturing of musculature, fat tissue and skin to my assistant. I step away from the table, leave the sterile area, get out of my gloves and the bloodied gown and call the patient's relatives from the OR as promised. Then I write the operation report. Even though the patient is still deep under anesthesia, he may notice this. Very little is known about where patients sojourn when they are asleep in the OR.

I imagine how tensely the relatives are waiting for my call. They shake and worry, and in my opinion every minute counts. While physically we may have treated only the patient's heart, we have touched a few more hearts indirectly, namely those of all the people who are connected with this patient through love, affection and worry. They are important, they are part of this, and with their help he will get better more quickly.

"Hello, this is Dr. Natour, am I speaking with Mrs. Schwarz?"

"Yes!"

I recognize her voice. She was present for the preoperative conversation.

"We are finished now. Your husband is stable. We did three bypasses, as discussed. There were no problems. We are transferring him to ICU now. I don't expect any issues and hope he will be awake in two or three hours. You can come around 5pm. If he is not yet awake then, you can still touch him a little. Or else you can call tonight. Then if you visit him tomorrow, he will look better as the tubes will be gone."

"And it's true that everything went well?"

"Yes, everything went according to plan."

It isn't always as straightforward as it was with Mr. Schwarz. Sometimes the vessels are bad, the bypass doesn't work properly. We can see how a heart attack might occur. Then I have to say something like: "We installed three bypasses, but one of them isn't looking too good. I don't yet know how things will develop. Hopefully it'll be okay."

In this way, I prepare the relatives for complications. It would be wrong to give them a false sense of security.

Before an operation is officially declared finished, we need to get through the sign-out – another checklist. We count: are all compresses there? Is the weight of the instruments, right? How much did they weigh before the operation, how much do they weigh after? In this way we can be sure that no scissors have been left inside the patient.

Were there any problems with the machines or instruments during the intervention?

Has the loss of blood been documented?

Has the postoperative care for the wound and the drains been discussed?

Has it been discussed how the patient has to be mobilized after the operation?

Have all procedures been documented?

Has the protocol for blood clotting, pain medication and antibiotics after the operation been discussed?

Has team communication been addressed? Are there any suggestions to improve the team's cooperation?

All colleagues know that after the operation there is time for these questions. In this way, no one has to think about them during the operation and everyone can totally focus on their work. There are some further points in the sign-out checklist, for example the question if all team members are listed in the protocol. The number of door movements is discussed; it should be as low as possible because of the risk of infection. Many small matters weave a safety net for the patients. The list is much longer still, but I will leave it at this.

I wish for such a safety net both preoperatively and postoperatively, so that the patients will not fall through as soon as they leave hospital and rehab. Figuratively speaking, we can "feed them up" in a way that they will become too big for that to happen.

Death on the Table

After the operation, we place the patient in his bed with all of their tubes and monitoring machines. Then I take them to the ICU. I rolled them into the OR, and now I'm rolling them out again. In most cases.

It is very rare that a patient dies during the operation. If it happens, it is extremely onerous for the whole team. A black cloud descends upon us. In the Netherlands, we take a lot of time to process it in the team. Everyone describes their impressions. There are situations in which it was foreseeable, for example with an aorta torn to tatters after a car accident. But routine procedures, too, can end in disaster. The system which is in place to help staff in such situations is better in the Netherlands than in Germany, in my opinion.

The conversation with the relatives after a patient's death sometimes goes similar to a preoperative talk in cases when we had to operate immediately, without a warning. The relatives are not receptive due to shock. They may ask why and how, but they are unable to process this information. That is why I offer a second meeting in a few weeks' time. Then they may arrive with a list, being ready for information about the operation. For many people it is very important to be able to comprehend everything, but not so much for others who think he/she is dead, why should I look into the reasons when they are not coming back.

It is often difficult to name the reasons. Some things work with one patient, but not with another – and we do not know why that is. It reminds us that we are human beings, not gods. A death always brings me back down to earth. Sure, my team and I have saved many lives. But not all of them.

If one has built a personal relationship with a patient, their death hurts even more. On the other hand, such a relationship helps me establish contact with their family. I know exactly who we are talking about; it was not a sick heart lined by green drapes, but a human being who was happy when working in the garden, helped many children with their homework as a volunteer and could tell jokes in a unique fashion.

The reactions of relatives to a patient's death are unpredictable. No one has ever reproached me. Once a teenage daughter pummeled me, despairingly and weakly; her pain needed an outlet, and I was the one standing next to her. She apologized the next day.

I know many colleagues – I'd say it is most of them – who prefer to avoid or delegate such conversations, or if indeed it must be done, they keep them as short as possible. For me, though, they are part of my job; they mark an end, different to the normal one that would see me accompany the patient to ICU: instead, I must deliver the news of a loved one's death.

I deem it important that we provide the relatives with names of people they can talk to in such a situation. There is a lot to say about grief, but I would like to turn back to the living soon, so let it suffice to mention that nowadays there is very good support for someone in mourning. I would wish this to be pointed out to every relative who loses a loved one in hospital so that they can be supported during the first steps of their mourning.

Sometimes patients whose operation has been successful grieve, too – they have lost something after all. In the worst case – which should for them be a stroke of luck – their old heart; or it could be a heart valve, or the feeling of being "intact", or living an untroubled life. For no apparent reason, some patients are deeply sad for weeks after an operation. They may not tell anyone as they are ashamed: everyone is happy as the operation went so well, but they feel this profound grief deep inside them. "I feel cut off from myself", one patient once told me. "As if I had lost a part of me during the operation."

We want to investigate such phenomena at our clinic, as we can help other patients when we know more. Maybe they will feel less alone then – you usually keep such strange thoughts to yourself: "Oh, there is such a thing? Oh, that's 'normal'? What a relief!"

First of all, though, the operation is followed by a critical phase. The procedure is done, but the patient is not out of the woods yet. Many things can still go wrong. The first twenty-four hours are especially dangerous. It is always an awful moment when I get to the clinic in the morning to find that a patient on whom I operated with my team the day before has died. I met the patient, they trusted me, we have walked a considerable part of their life's path together, in some way they have become a part of me. I left the clinic last night with a good feeling; maybe the patient whom I had operated on in the morning was awake when I looked in on them. But they had to be reanimated in the night, and we lost them. When that happens, it is terrible.

Sometimes I get a second chance. I am called, maybe because a secondary bleeding was detected. In a great rush I drive to the clinic, where the patient is already being prepared – and then I operate again, trying to close the leakage. As this can happen now and then, it is important not to give the relatives a false sense of security, but instead to remind them after the operation that the climb is still a steep one.

If the mountain cannot be climbed, my role changes in the eyes of the relatives; the former savior becomes a perpetrator. Before I interfered, the husband was alive. The patient dies because I operated on him. Without the operation, he may have died the next day, or the one after that – but the fact is that he died during the procedure. While I did not kill him – he bled to death – it affects me, even though I know I am not to blame. As a surgeon I experience the same steps in the graph (see above at the end of the chapter OPENING) as my patients. I am fine when an operation is successful. If things go wrong, I crash.

You can never know in advance what exactly will happen. None of the preliminary examinations can really tell us what to expect when we open the thorax, or how the patient's body will react to the enormity of this event.

In Germany, all patients who die during an operation are treated as deaths from unnatural causes. The police will be informed, the corpse will be confiscated, and a forensic autopsy arranged. This can put additional strain on the relatives. In the Netherlands, an autopsy will be performed on a deceased patient only if the family wishes. For doctors, an autopsy is always a chance to learn something; therefore, I would like more positive responses to requests for autopsies. Causes will come to light which we cannot guess, for example a thrombosis of the intestinal vessels. Thromboses, meaning coagulation disorders, are a great risk during heart surgery, as we are disturbing the circulation, change the blood's density for the heart-lung machine, making it thinner and then thicker again. On top of that, we install foreign materials such as a heart valve or a prosthesis. Sometimes we see clots forming during an operation – which we of course dissolve; yet once a patient is closed up again, we no longer have access.

I must shake off a death on the table as quickly as possible. In the Netherlands, we get a "grace period" of one day. A colleague will take over our next operation. The rest is simply professionalism you acquire over the years. It would be desirable for students to be better prepared for situations like this.

In my opinion there are too few obligatory courses during a degree in medicine which convey to aspiring medical professionals the situation of patients and relatives. We need seminars in which we grapple with the things that will happen to us as medics when we cross the border between life and death and when something goes wrong. I consider it wrong to claim that it is only the psychologists who should look after the soul. The soul is part of the medical degree! I want doctors to deal with this without fear; death, after all, is our greatest enemy.

Farewells

The fear of death is so central to our existence that many philosophers view it as the origin of religion, art, culture, and science. From a psychological point of view, one of the biggest human achievements is fighting off the thought of our own death. According to some psychologists, preventing thoughts of our own death is a main function of human perception, action, and self-knowledge.

Furthermore, our society suppresses death. In our everyday life in Western society, we are only rarely confronted with death. People in Western societies lose a close relative approximately every fifteen years. In former times – and in many parts of the world also today – death was omnipresent, and it was mainly younger people who died: infants, children, youth, mothers, soldiers. They died from hunger, illness, epidemics, wars, insufficient medical treatment, and catastrophic hygienic conditions.

In the past, death was predominantly quick, often by infections. Today we often die slowly and over a long period of time. That is true especially for older people with advanced cancer and other chronic illnesses.

Death was formerly a familiar companion. Family, friends, and neighbors would spend the last hours by the dying person's bedside. They prayed together and said farewell together. They washed and dressed the deceased together and prepared them for the public viewing. Then the relatives and friends again sat with them when keeping vigil. This could last for several days, and the coffin was carried or driven openly through the village before the funeral.

Today the coffins are banned from the streets, and some funeral homes remove anything that could identify their vehicle as a hearse. That makes it easier for us to deal with illness, death and dying. The dead and dying are removed from everyday life and handed over to professionals "for processing". As a result, people have increased insecurity in dealing with death and dying. In my childhood and youth, illness and death were a natural part of life. Occasionally there were people who were sick and needed help; we supported them without giving much thought to it. There weren't any rest homes in my childhood; the families cared for their older relatives. I am sure that no dead person would have remained undetected in their apartment for weeks. Someone would probably have missed them the very next day.

As I mentioned, I practice in two countries. They sometimes envy me in Germany, along the lines of the system is much better in the Netherlands, where doctors do not have to keep the dying alive. A doctor is not committing a crime when they help end a life which has lost all dignity. But I do not want to be a service provider for transport into death. Firstly, there is palliative care. Secondly – and this is important to me– we should not let our society drift into a state where the old and the sick are first pushed into rest homes and then handed over to hospitals they won't ever leave again – as if that would satisfy everyone. In my opinion, if someone does not want to be a burden on anyone and thus wishes to part with this life voluntarily, that is the declaration of defeat of a society which only values those who can perform. Which future do we want to live in? We are shaping it today.

Death nowadays is often before our eyes on a screen – it is virtual, not of flesh and blood. Few have seen "real" dead people, maybe parents or grandparents, lying on the bed as if asleep; but we see thousands on TV. To avoid death does not work. Those who do not say good-bye to someone who has died, because they want to remember them as they were, do themselves a disservice in many cases.

A farewell is always a full stop, an end. Even if it is extremely painful, it ends a chapter, and a new one begins. It has been proven that those mourners who can say farewell to their dead continue their lives with a better and more secure feeling and go through the natural phases of grieving without traumatic breakdowns.

Children, too, can be brought along to a final farewell, independent of their age. You should not talk them into it, though – they should wish to come along of their own accord. You can encourage them to choose a toy for the dead person or to draw a picture for grandma or granddad or brother or sister, which then will be put in the coffin. Such acts are important; we give the dear departed something to take with them.

Ideally, however, we accompany our loved ones on the path back to life – which starts in the intensive care unit.

12

INTENSIVELY UNCONSCIOUS

A person in ICU cannot survive without high-tech medicine. They are not conscious of this; in hindsight, the stay in ICU seems like a nebulous time for many patients.

Standing by the sickbed of Richard Schwarz, I hand my patient over to the team in ICU. While he will be connected to various monitoring machines, I recount not only his medical history but also say a few sentences about him. I think it is nice to hand over not just a patient but also a human being.

However, what is most important for the handover are the medical details. No information must be missing, so that no disaster can develop from any small matter. We have strained his circulation considerably, shut down his heart and cooled down his body. The patient is still cool when he arrives in ICU, even though we warmed up his blood again at the end of the operation. It will take some time for the temperature to stabilize – and as his vessels will widen while this happens, there is a certain risk. Secondary bleedings and many other problems may also occur. In ICU, the patient is in the best hands and under constant surveillance. And that is the moment when I say good-bye to him.

I look forward to a break, to finally sit down after standing at the table for many hours, put my feet up, drink something. In the clinic in Oldenburg, surgeons had thirty minutes between two operations. My current university clinic grants me more time.

How long a patient remains in ICU depends on their condition. A favorable development can already see them transferred to a normal ward on the day after the operation. Or else it can take a while because the wound won't heal well, or other complications come up. When secondary bleedings occur, we must operate again, which of course disrupts the surgery schedule.

We gently reduce the anesthetics while patients wake up. We watch them very closely. Some are very confused, agitated, try to pull the drips from their body. Usually, they wake up when their pulmonary status is okay and their circulation is stable, and neither secondary bleedings nor arrhythmia have occurred. When the patients are able to cough, mobilizing phlegm, the breathing tube is also removed. The patients normally don't notice this; if they do, it is very unpleasant.

Before I leave the clinic in the evening, I look in on my patient again.

"How are you feeling, Mr. Schwarz?"

"Well."

"I'm glad."

"I'm so happy that it's behind me now."

"I believe you", I reply, hoping that the worst is indeed behind him. I look in on other patients, too.

"How are you feeling, Mrs. Lange?", I ask.

Her response is whispered: "I have to buy milk."

This response shows me that this patient is in a transitory postoperative delirium. This is an intermediate state, marked by disorientation. A layperson can imagine this as the slow reduction of the different pain medication and anesthetic.

Transitory Postoperative Delirium

Normally patients have met me before the operation. When they are in a postoperative delirium, they often no longer know who I am. They are not master or mistress of their senses and do not know they are in ICU. They may indeed wrongly believe they are in another country at another time while they are speaking with a nurse or their relatives. This phenomenon has different causes, and medical research has not yet reached any final conclusion. It is as if the patient were living in a parallel world.

New attempt.

"Hello Mrs. Lange", I greet my patient. "How are you feeling?"

"I have to hurry", she says. "Otherwise, I will miss the train."

"Mrs. Lange, you are in intensive care at the clinic in Maastricht."

"What nonsense."

"My name is Dr. Natour, and I operated on your heart four days ago."

"Get out of my way, I'm in a hurry, I have to catch my train."

In her imagination, this patient is not lying helplessly in her bed but is in a train station.

"Mrs. Lange, we are in the intensive care unit here."

"I don't believe you." Her eyes wander through the room. I don't know what she is seeing; it is definitely not a patient's room, as she is insisting on having to go to her train now. And then she falls asleep. Where will she be when she wakes up? Will she have arrived then?

In reality, it will always be this room. Not an airport, nor a shopping center. Patients told me that they had been put into a different bed every day, or that we have to observe better hygiene in the hospital as there are white mice scurrying everywhere. White mice are strangely popular. When three different patients tell you about white mice one after another, you start to wonder at some point who is right. But a delirium is no funny matter. It is a psychotic state, and patients often experience severe anxiety, panic attacks and the resurfacing of past traumas. We noticed that patients who are very afraid before the intervention are at a greater risk in this regard than the less fearful ones. This shows again how important good preparation can be.

In a postoperative delirium, patients fall out of time and space. An older patient did not dare to breathe – fearing for her life, she was afraid that the soldiers who were looking for her would find and kill her. She was not in her ICU bed in 2021, but in World War II. Other patients believed to be in torture chambers, in hell, living through the most horrible situations or witnessing their family's death.

If this transitional stage with all its highs and lows were better known generally, the patients and their relatives and friends could make better sense of it. As it is, it creates a lot of anxiety for many relatives who fear it will now be like this forever; but it is the patients in the first instance who are deeply unsettled by these psychotic episodes. Often, they cannot confide in anyone because they worry they will be thought crazy. They ask themselves if madness will recur and where they can find the exit to reality – and even: what *is* real? What I believe, no, more than that: what I *know*? Or what they want me to believe in here?

When their minds become clearer step by step, they forget a lot or even everything. Others who can remember may be very irritated, especially those who are usually the down-to-earth types in whose life imagination never played a role. A filmmaker was once positively enthusiastic about the "great show" she had experienced. She is an exception though because the screenplays are usually not nice. The worst is when patients believe – and that happens often – to be kidnapped and tortured. They see their relatives talk to the nursing staff and want to signal that the nurses are really torturers, but can't get the words out. Everyone can imagine what sort of hell those patients live through.

It is a dilemma for the nursing staff, too. We want to help, but we are pushed away, insulted, treated badly. A patient in ICU does not have much strength, but it is not nice to work in an environment where the care of patients is misconstrued as an attack on their life and limb. An added issue is that patients with postoperative delirium often require additional nursing efforts. They may pull drips from their body so that sometimes they must be restrained as intravenous therapy is jeopardized; they fall out of their bed because they believe to have to urgently get to the train or elsewhere, or they think that a pursuer is breathing down their neck. They may injure themselves in the process. An awful lot of understanding and patience is required of the nurses – and it is generally known that many hospital wards are stretched to their limit, even with just the "normal" nursing requirements.

Why do we make it so difficult for both ourselves and the patients? That really is not what we want, of course not. The practical constraints are to blame. Who creates those? Let's say we are responsible for them – in which case we could ease them, could we not?

"Mr. Richter, you are in hospital. Mr. Richter, please, you must not pull on the drains. You had heart surgery." Mr. Richter does not believe a word. And three white mice are running again... why doesn't anyone see them? Is he surrounded by a bunch of mad people here?

The duration of a delirium depends on its cause and especially on its severity. Older patients are affected more often and longer. Contact with their relatives can build a bridge to reality. That requires, though, for the relatives to be well prepared to deal with a patient in delirium. It is counterproductive for them to repeat mantra-like that there are no white mice. Sensitive communication is called for; then again, they should not pretend to see white mice, too.

Sometimes there is a click, and someone is back again.

Sometimes they return in small steps. And they might be embarrassed when they are told what they said and did. It should definitely not be brought up again and again or even turned into an anecdote: *imagine, he has...* That would remind the patient permanently of this terrible loss of control.

Many people soon have only a vague memory of this in-between world. Yet when it surfaces, they should know that it is normal. It is part of the process. It is nothing to be ashamed about. We should explain this to them beforehand, so that it becomes easier later. It is part of their recovery. And now they have pulled through. Onward to their new normal they go.

13

BACK TO MY
OLD SELF?

To an extent, patients still feel wrapped in cotton wool when they are transferred to a normal ward. By and by the drains come out, there is more to eat than just mashed-up food, they may be able to eat without any assistance, will soon manage to go to the toilet using their rolling walker, then without it, and their cheeks get some color back.

The normal ward is the waiting room for normal life. At this stage, the patients feel safe and secure in the medical care they receive. They are full of hope to soon be their old self again. Some feel how exhausted they are and how little they are capable of. They suffer from different discomforts; throat aches caused by the anesthesia are common, they can't swallow properly. Slowly it dawns on them that the operation and the transfer out of ICU means they have come a part of the road, but that the finish line is still far away. Some patients are disheartened by this realization because they don't know where to find the strength to reach that finish line. Others are motivated by the prospect of taking responsibility for themselves and their lives again.

After an operation involving a heart-lung machine, about thirty percent of patients experience arrhythmia, or more specifically atrial fibrillation, which may cause a very alarming feeling and great fear. When one just had a heart operation…*is something wrong? Is this dangerous? Is a heart attack looming?* The patients listen to what is going on inside them; some lie in their beds as if paralyzed, hardly daring to breathe. They put their body into preservation mode, take only shallow breaths – which is the worst they can do; this is why respiratory exercises should be started early. Ideally, several therapists visit the patients in the normal ward. Patients should internalize how important it is for their recovery to be active, to participate and continue to do the recommended exercises once they are back at home.

This applies to any crisis. Stay alert! Be proactive! After all, to have survived one crisis does not mean there won't be another – the next one can be right outside the door.

It is best for the patients to get addresses and tips when they are still in the clinic, for example for a cardiac rehab group. Sure, a clinic is not a place for aftercare, but it should be initiated and actively started here; tips for the different possibilities should be provided from the beginning, even during the preoperative conversation, so that the patients realize that they have a long road with various stages in front of them.

As the trust in one's body and abilities are often in

a sorry state, it is now vital to build up their mental strength. This means to not constantly advise them how to tread carefully, but to encourage them: "Your body is strong. You have come so far, you will master the next stages, too." Occupational therapists and others can provide valuable support in this phase. There are many supporting measures between physiotherapy and psychotherapy. I think psychological support is always useful, as a sensitive phase begins after a patient's discharge from the clinic and later rehab, when it will become obvious how well they master their everyday life. They will find their way back into life more easily the better prepared they are, the more strategies they have learned, the better they understand that changes are normal, and the more they see that they can share such changes with their social environment. Part of this is knowing upfront that they will never fully be their old self again but a new self.

Listening to what is going on inside them can take up a lot of space for the patients. It can go so far that they develop fears about having to manage without medical support. Something bad could happen – what then? The patients are weak and have little faith in themselves. It is enormously important to give them a positive outlook: they will not have to live as a patient forever but will be able to shape their life again on their own authority and free of fear. The relatives, for whom such a life is largely the norm, should understand that the returnees are starting from scratch. Maybe they will join in and find new rituals together with the patients.

Flying Visit at Home

If everything goes according to plan, the patient will

be discharged five or six days after the operation. Some long for this day to arrive, while it comes as a surprise for others. It depends on what is waiting for the patient at home. If they are alone, can they take care of themselves, or do they need help? Are they longingly expected by a caring family? Or is the family worried they may not be up to the task? Even though there may be no medical reasons not to discharge a patient, some of them still seem very needy. They lie in their bed during ward round, merely managing to feebly lift their hand, signaling that they need a little more time. In the end, the doctors decide; if we can take the responsibility for a discharge from a medical point of view, there will be no postponement – sometimes also because we need the bed urgently.

Other patients in the same situation sit upright in their bed at ward round time and leave no doubt that they want out.

I have noticed that it makes a difference for both sides if we encounter a lying patient or a sitting one. When they sit, they are more at eye level with us: they invite more respect and attention. Patients lying down will be overlooked more easily, and their dignity is also hurt when they are talked about, and decisions are made on their behalf. Patient sitting on the edge of their bed have straightened themselves up, wanting to be taken seriously; they display more courage and responsibility – and thus feel much better about themselves.

The discharge usually means only a flying visit at home. Every patient is entitled to physical rehabilitation, and most indeed complete such a program. Occasionally, patients go straight from the clinic to rehab, but usually they are at home first for a few days. These days are a test for the time after rehab. Many sensitivities may arise, as the patients leave a protected zone when they get out of the clinic. Supposing they came to the clinic as a relatively healthy person on their own two feet, they will leave as a patient, maybe in a wheelchair or on very wobbly feet. A wife brought her husband to the hospital and now brings a patient home.

Many become aware of this now, but don't discuss it openly – it hurts too much. How do patients deal with it? Will they try by hook or by crook to at least play the role of their old self, even though they are no longer that person and it requires a tremendous effort to pretend? Or will they rather remain in their protected zone, constantly reminding those around them that they need a lot of care? Or do those around them believe that the patients will have to be fussed over all the time, which can become annoying to the recovering patients as they feel as if their brain had been operated on rather than their heart? And when they respond angrily, those who had their best interests in mind feel hurt.

Sometimes relatives are afraid to be at home alone with the patient, without medical support. In this situation it helps if one has noted down all important telephone numbers and steps to take in an emergency – or if one even packs a bag to have it handy when there is the justified worry that another stay in hospital might become necessary.

For relatives to understand the diagnosis and the ensuing course of action can be useful, as it means that they come along to medical appointments and ask questions of the doctors, even though they are affected only indirectly. Psychological support for relatives should be a matter of course. The aim is to take the horror out of the illness and understand it as well as all necessary changes that will now have to be made, particularly at the beginning. Is a special bed needed, which medication will need to be taken, are there any dietary requirements, and so on? Obviously, it is all very exhausting for the relatives – and it is no surprise that at times they will feel drained and then have a bad conscience because they are the healthy ones.

A relative once told me that when she was overwhelmed, she sometimes imagined that her husband was not there at all anymore. In this way, she was then able to care for him with a lot of calmness and patience.

There are distinct patterns which can come to the fore at this stage. They follow psychological "screenplays". It is a great relief to know them. One such screenplay shows us a stressed wife who realized in her husband's absence how much easier things go for her without him. Ultimately, she feels it would be better if he didn't return to her. But one must not even think something like that, let alone say it aloud. She knows that her feelings for him have cooled down, yet she will have to help him a lot for some time to come. Things have always been done his way; matters always have had to center on him. And now everything is about him again, but this time he cannot help it. Can he really not help it? Or has he brought this upon himself with his lifestyle, and she is to pull him out?

In another screenplay we meet a patient who has family matters considerately and firmly under control. He always looks after everything and everyone. A veritable patriarch. Authoritarian, but also bighearted – tough on the outside, soft on the inside. Everyone is used to him calling the shots. He feels nothing short of obliged to pretend he is still calling them. He does not know any different role. No one in this family knows any other role. I am thinking of a specific patient for this screenplay, who had the courage to one day say to his wife: "I can't manage anymore." In that moment, she realized that he was no longer his old self and probably would never be again. Compared to many others in such a situation, she felt no fear but saw it as a chance. It was of great importance, though, for the patriarch to abdicate – for him to show weakness to make the family strong again.

If there are children in the family, this always creates a situation which is particularly fragile, as they urgently need stability. It can unsettle them greatly if one parent becomes severely ill. That has consequences for the healthy parent as well, and thus children lose their safe base. In such cases, we should consider if someone else can help out for a while. While a patient goes through aftercare, it is advisable – maybe with psychological support – to make sure that the children have overcome the crisis well. Grown-up children, too, can lose their footing when their parents are ailing. If there are siblings, they often display completely different coping strategies. There is the thirty-year-old son who will not visit the father in hospital as he is unable to bear his helplessness, while the younger daughter finds a proper connection to him for the first time in this situation. There may be quarrels within the family as to who will take on which tasks. Alliances are formed, the system is on its head, new roles must be found. In this way, a crisis is also an opportunity for everyone involved to surprise themselves, to get to know new sides of their own personalities, to mature overall.

A further screenplay shows a family or a relationship in which emotions are rarely talked about, along the lines of: I once told you that I love you, and that should be enough until life's end. Worry and anxiety are among the concealed emotions. If they are not articulated, they sometimes come out in a weird way. I remember a husband who after his wife's operation – certainly also fueled by COVID-19 – became a veritable hygiene fanatic. He not only drove his wife crazy with his hygiene rules, but his whole family and friends – who he would have liked to keep away from his wife altogether as he saw them only as spreaders of the virus. She felt harassed by him until she saw his motive for what it was: loving care, fear for his beloved wife. From that moment, his behavior was no longer an imposition but a proof of love. That said, it took a bit of crisis intervention until the husband put the responsibility for his wife's health back where it belonged – into her hands.

With female patients I sometimes notice that their relatives are so used to them taking care of the whole family with such self-sacrifice, that it does not even occur to them to go easy on the person who is now a patient. A mother doesn't "drop out", she is always available! She herself is convinced of this and does not want to show that she can no longer muster the necessary strength. Women like this haven't learned to look after themselves and take their needs seriously. Now – they will have to learn it, as do their relatives.

It may also be that relatives are underappreciated. The phone rings constantly, with someone asking: "How is he/she?" Nobody asks after the relatives. They make sure that everything remains stable, they are on their feet morning to night to the point of exhaustion – but they are deemed irrelevant.

Furthermore, there is the fact that the patients, who

often have many needs after their operation, also desire company. They wish to talk, have their hand held, they want attention and may enjoy being taken care of. Usually, these demands vanish once patients become more independent; the relatives should have that in mind. Many studies show, by the way, that patients who feel comforted and supported by others are better able to handle their symptoms and may even recover more quickly.

Relatives can contribute a lot to the shaping of their time together with the patients. While they are not doctors, they can make sure that the mood is good. For that to happen, however, they need to be in control of themselves and their impulses. In a good relationship, the patient's partners are sometimes positively animated by the chance to now spoil their loved one. How we treat each other today is the result of how we treated each other yesterday. Some relationships will not withstand the strain of a serious illness; for other relationships it may lead to a reinvigoration.

It is crucial that relatives, apart from all the love and help they give, do not forget to look after themselves – after all, many others forget them already. Take care of yourself. Free up time for yourself. You are not a bad person if you need a break – and these breaks should constitute a regular part of the daily and weekly plans. They are your time-outs during which you can gather strength. Get some support for yourself, too. Maybe a neighbor can take over the cooking, the bowling club might organize a trip, a nurse might come in the mornings and help with the washing, whatever it may be. If you delegate, you show competence, intelligence, and strong leadership.

Relationship patterns become obvious during crisis situations. Old balances no longer work; we have a chance to reshuffle the cards. This is an attitude I want to promote with our foundation. The earlier we prepare for the fact that things will never again be as they were before, the better the chances will be for all of us. The relatives play a decisive role at this stage in the patient's life. To talk to each other is key; when we cannot communicate our worries, fear, resentment, and love because we are afraid to hurt the partner or make them angry, these emotions will manifest in some other way. We should not expect too much of ourselves. We are all human. Depending on how we feel on a particular day, we manage to muster understanding for another person's situation with different levels of success. We must also remember the fact that patients are thin-skinned and sensitive after a severe intervention. Their relatives don't know them like this. Some of them fear that this sensitivity will remain forever; usually, though, it vanishes once the patient gains more belief in themselves. It may also be lovely to discover new character traits in a person we have known for a long time. If we are not afraid of this, profound new encounters may happen.

Relatives can help patients come to terms with their illness in four different ways. Firstly, through emotional support, consolation, and care. Secondly, through practical assistance, for example handling daily chores or transport. Thirdly, there is financial support, and fourthly, advice and help with finding information. Every person is different. Not everyone requires the same level of support, which means that we should first find out where exactly help is needed. Is the patient someone who has enough love and care, but does not cope with organizing their everyday life? Or is everything perfectly organized, but they feel lonely? Relatives may at times be over-motivated, or else they only help where they like to help. We need to leave our comfort zone to provide the help which is necessary in a crisis. By giving support where it is required, we make sure that the crisis will be managed well. This is also the aim of rehab.

My Fate is Not Unique: Rehab

Not everyone is looking forward to their rehab. For many, it is a necessary evil. How they would like to stay at home, finally immersing themselves in their normal life again. Sociability makes rehab easier, as one will meet strangers. One can also do rehab as an outpatient; however, if one decides to do that in order to start helping around one's home again, it is not advisable – because in rehab you should be completely focused on recovery and recreation. Furthermore, rehab is often a good place to find interesting information about financial aspects, pensions, and other government benefits. Rehab is, by law, designed to remove the "impairment of one's capacity to work", or prevent or postpone "the early exit from the workforce".

The word "rehabilitation" comes from the Latin and means to restore or re-enable someone. In a medical sense, it means that the original state of someone's health is to be re-established for the benefit of their personal, social, and professional life. However, that is not always successful. Many patients will experience limitations after an operation, while others will experience an improvement, for example after a heart valve operation: they will breathe more easily and are more productive overall.

Rehab aims to make everyday things possible, to build self-confidence and independence, and to regain one's quality of life. Not infrequently former patients who initially felt reluctant about rehab are in the end very happy to have completed it. It is another tense period on their way back to their old life. They are no longer patients, but also not yet fully restored. Rehab builds them a bridge back to their life, which they can use with relatively good mobility.

Surrounded by people who also have fallen out of life, so to speak, you meet fellow sufferers with similar fates in rehab. How do they deal with it? Some are worse off than you, others had more luck. You hear stories, learn from each other, hear new things, get good tips, tell your own story, and can incorporate the recent past: I'm the one with the new valve. I'm the one with the scar. I'm the one with the accident. I'm the one with the burnout etc. This is enormously important as you can't deny what has happened and will bring this change to your everyday life. Surrounded by fellow sufferers, it may be easier to talk about some things from which you want to protect your relatives. Relatives and friends often do not know what really goes on inside the heads of former patients. How are they supposed to imagine it? Here in rehab people share similar experiences and often feel understood – if they use the opportunity, that is.

Unfortunately, some patients withdraw and merely wait for it to be over. That is a pity. If someone only strives to leave it all behind as quickly as possible, they miss many opportunities that could help them. We observe, for example, that patients do not make use of the proffered conversations with psychologists; especially those who never had dealings with a psychologist and self-diagnose: "I'm sure I don't need a psychiatrist" could gain a whole new perspective. In our foundation *Stilgezet*, we want to arouse patients' curiosity about these opportunities so that they can use them without prejudice.

Rehab is still part of the phase of convalescence. Some uncertainties can be worked out at this time. There are numerous therapeutic treatments and medical care, but it is not a hospital. There are set times for scheduled activities, but patients can also do things by themselves. Patients often marvel at their progress in rehab. Some notice an improvement after just a few days. From a physiological point of view, the body needs a few weeks to six months until it is out of the woods – if all goes well, that is. The time depends on the nature of the intervention: a heart valve operation is absorbed more quickly than a big repair of the aorta.

Patients ask again and again how long it will take – it is already a topic during the preoperative conversation. The self-employed particularly often feel high pressure to be able to work again as fast as possible, even more so if they are a family's sole earner. After the operation they realize that it will take them considerably longer than they had hoped. They barely manage a few steps when they climb stairs – how will they acquire new customers given their breathlessness and disastrous mental state? They experience an exhaustion, a tiredness, a profound feebleness which they had never thought possible. Some did not notice it when they were in hospital, as they lay in their bed a lot. But now, when they should be mobile, it becomes frighteningly clear to them how worn out they are. Even the sporty types may be glad to manage to sit on a stool during physiotherapy. For some, this decline in fitness causes a depressive mood. They do not see any light at the end of the tunnel, and they despair. Others become angry or impatient. Secretly they are afraid that this weakness will never pass. Some withdraw completely and do not want to talk to anyone. Others need the exchange of stories, especially with those who have attended rehab for a while already and can tell them: "My first week was a disaster, but look, now I can already swim three lanes without a break. Believe me, you will get better, too. Be patient!"

Doctors can only remind patients again and again that their body has gone through something unbelievable, although it is not visible from the outside. If the wound heals well, soon only a scar will be visible. Hence the patients forget their ordeal, or else they cannot or do not want to imagine it. But their body was cut open, its inner layout changed. The body is not a living room where you move a few pieces of furniture, and then they just stand somewhere else, done. Everything in the body that was cut will have to grow together again. Maybe the idea of designing a garden can help you don't sow on a Monday in March, and on Tuesday everything is in full bloom. It takes time. It will be even more beautiful in May.

Some patients feel as if they have been emptied completely and then filled again with everything in the wrong spot. "When I take a breath, my hearts hits the sternum." They speak of drumming against their chest. Everything feels tense. Nothing is right anymore. And always shortness of breath. The body feels strange. "I feel like a stranger inside myself." Some tell of a stabbing pain when they breathe, like a knife in the lungs or abdomen. They are afraid to breathe deeply and accustom themselves to shallow breathing, which can result in pneumonia as the lungs are not properly ventilated. This means leaving rehab and going back into hospital. A terrible setback, which could have been avoided if the patients had been better informed from the outset about what to pay attention to after the operation and why.

In my experience, my patients will participate very well if they understand the context. That may take five extra minutes of explanation but will later prevent weeks of a difficult recovery. Breathing exercises should be included as a matter of course especially after operations concerning the upper body. The thorax will of course hurt where the drain was. Yet to tread too softly is the wrong approach. With professional guidance, the patients learn to breathe beyond the point when pain occurs, so that they regain breathing space, ventilate the lungs well and in general feel better with a good oxygen supply.

Often people in rehab are so focused on their body that they do not manage to care for the soul, which according to experience requires more time and sometimes comes forward crestfallen: "Why me? Why do I have to put up with all this? How can I go on? Will those on the outside ever take me seriously?"

The relatives see someone who was gone. Now they come back. They should be who they always were. But how can one explain that one has become a different person? Ideally, the patient will befriend this new version of themselves during rehab. Resolutions are made frequently, and sometimes the brainstorm hits at this point already: maybe all this rubbish had something good to it, too – as a new beginning.

The relatives ask: "How are you, are you feeling better,

do you really believe you'll be able to work again soon, do you think we can go on vacation this summer?"

They give encouragement: "It will be okay, you have to be patient, we'll manage."

Sometimes they despair, maybe because they have a business with their partner, and they signal: "I don't know how I'm meant to manage all this by myself."

In this case, the person in rehab will comfort the visitor. Maybe they notice that the relatives show less understanding for them now than they did during the hospital stay. In their minds, the worst is over. The operation was successful. Now, if you don't mind, things can return to normal. In such a situation, it would be helpful if the relatives, too, get another explanation of what goes on with the patient's body now. Occasionally, it is the relatives who remind the patient of this – who pretends that nothing has happened. On some, it dawns now that they are still far away from calm waters. The patient recounts on the phone: "Today I went up the stairs to the first floor without taking a break." What a success! At home, there are three floors without a lift. Will they manage that?

"When I'm back at home, we will go to the swimming pool every Saturday morning. What do you think?", the patient asked her husband.

"Into the water that early? No thanks."

It would be nice if the family back at home could seize the impulses which the patient brings from rehab. Relationship patterns show again. How do I deal with the new things my partner wants to incorporate into the relationship? Do I reject everything on principle, or am I happy about how this may liven up the place? And if not: why on earth not?

I often hear that patients feel paralyzed or like they don't belong anywhere. They feel as if they are benched, removed from the game of life, always observed, and eyeballed by the caring relatives. Is everything okay? Maybe the relatives are very anxious – nothing must go wrong, please. Things must become as they were. They keep their worries to themselves but may react gruffly because they need to take on more than before. Or else they are overprotective, which leads to the patients having less confidence, feeling weaker and sicker than they are – and in the worst case they might never properly get back on their feet. Honesty is extremely important during this sensitive phase, even if taboos are broken. Psychology starts to play a role. Does a wife want to exchange her husband for a patient? He in turn will become grumpy, angry – he is not a patient, not him, he is still a real man. This drives the wife to despair, as he should take it easy. I know some women who administrate their husbands' illness – who themselves pay it no mind at all. Then I know patients who after a "big deal" demand to be constantly wrapped in cotton wool. Many are afraid once they leave the shelter that is the hospital and rehab. No doctor is constantly near them anymore. If something were to happen now... These thoughts are permanent reminders that there is no old normal, no normal at all.

Rehab offers protection from the outside world where normal life continues. Patients feel this distinction very clearly. At times they are happy when they get a glimpse of the outside, at others they are afraid.

"Will I be able to cope with everyday life? What do the others think about me? Will I be a burden for them? Does my wife/

husband still find me attractive? How can I show the children that I'm back now? Will I be laid off at work? Whom will I tell what exactly happened to me? Yes, whom do I trust? Do I really have that many friends? Or are they acquaintances rather? Strange, I feel closer to some people in here than to others on the outside whom I've known for so long. Will I be able to ski again?"

Questions come and go; depending on one's condition there are several answers – but the soul will have the last word, and when something is right, we feel it.

When people think about their lives in rehab and maybe re-arrange their value system, they often want to spend more time with their loved ones in the future. To be more attentive. To eat a healthier diet, get exercise – one's health is the most important thing after all. Maybe a wish from long ago comes to mind. As I child, I dreamed of Alaska. Or of a horse. Why not – a trip to Alaska and in the longer run start horse-riding again. Don't make so many appointments. To just drift on weekends. Read books. Stare into space. Go for a walk with one's love. Hand in hand. Have long breakfasts. Go to the movies. Simply do nice things. Be tender. Don't look so much at what the others have, more at what they are. Time for oneself. Reduce the speed.

Such a relaxed attitude to life is classified as inertia by a 24/7 society that rushes its members through the days and to which the concept of functioning is central. Curiously enough, there is an expectation at the same time that those who are asked to run around the clock should always be relaxed when doing so. A burn-out is something that only happens to fools.

When a patient realizes they can't continue to live like

they used to, they may feel superfluous – they are not achieving anything. How will their employer manage their reintegration? Will they be in danger of losing their job? You know how these things go. First operated on, then dismissed. To find a new job at age sixty is not easy, even more so as you would have to be convincing in an interview – when on the inside you are still weakened from your experience. In this way, an able employee will not infrequently be pushed aside.

Not everyone succeeds in developing a new perspective. Some feel badly treated after all they have done for the firm. Great disappointment sets in. One thought one was valued as a human being, and yet as soon as one no longer functions they discard you. Ready for the junkyard. In our experience, people often decline very quickly if they are not given a new chance. What a waste of resources, as these crisis survivors would have so much to offer!

Why do we not give the returnees more time so that they can test their limits and then continue to work at an appropriate level? Who says that a person in a leadership role must work fifty or more hours per week? Who makes these rules? Quantity does not equal quality.

Women's hearts deal better with such hardships – they are quicker to find alternatives and, generally speaking, do not tie their self-esteem to professional recognition. Men's hearts like to bottle up these hardships; they give up more easily, fight less and become passive.

In convalescence, too, we often find women to be fitter than men. Some men become completely dependent on their wives who, as already mentioned, administrate their health: what the husband may eat, when he takes which pills and so on. Such "strong men" stand in the kitchen of the house where they have lived for thirty years, asking completely overwhelmed: "Where are the pots? Do we have a cucumber slicer?" When they come home from rehab, and if their wife is at work, they worriedly ask how they might get a cup of coffee. In a restaurant, maybe? Or a neighbor will show mercy. It sounds strange, I know, but the "tough boys" from the last millennium are not extinct yet. Once a patient told me that she had pre-cooked and frozen fifty meals for her husband. Three weeks in the clinic plus three weeks rehab, she had calculated, plus a buffer in case the rehab took longer.

"How old is your husband?", I asked her, expecting to hear of a person well advanced in years and presumably severely ill.

"Sixty-two." She sighed. "But he is working the whole day and only comes home at six."

I nodded and studied her face to see if she had made a joke. No, she was being serious. While I stepped to the next bed, I wondered why she or his mother or anyone hadn't taught him how to cook. Or was it a good feeling for the patient to provide for her husband before her operation? Night after night he could defrost a meal and feel her love. Or did she enjoy his dependence on her, and did he enjoy it as well? Some men will remain tied to someone's apron strings their whole life.

When I think back to my childhood, my father was only ever working in the kitchen when my mother was in the clinic for three or four days to give birth to a sibling. There were many of those in our family, but I was looking forward to every new arrival. During this time my father looked after us, the work in the fields was on hold. I can see him before me still, standing in the kitchen. An unusual sight. I don't remember if his food was tasty, but I am sure we were all happy when mother was back home. And yes, I can cook, I even like it a lot. It relaxes me. I love to cook after a day of difficult procedures – from surgical tools to kitchen tools. Maybe we should offer cooking classes for some patients in rehab – after all it is the goal for the patients to manage their life at home. Part of this is to interrupt old patterns which could cause stress.

Various relaxation techniques are offered in rehab: autogenic training, progressive muscle relaxation, yoga, meditation. They all help to find the ground under one's feet again. It is crucial for some people to learn new ways of how to deal with their emotions – or else to gain access to their feelings and listen to their gut feeling in the first place. Emotions are frequently suppressed, including those related to the illness. It is enormously important to recognize and deal with them, so they don't make trouble below the surface. Feelings of guilt, for example, are very common. Yet how can a person be guilty of their illness – it would be as if I would call myself a bad father when one of my children gets up to no good.

As is often the case towards the end of a crisis, when the worst is behind us, we see quite clearly how we can avoid the next one. But will we take our resolutions to heart? How many crises are required before we can rouse ourselves to worry about prevention? That depends on our capacity for suffering or maybe our love of enjoyment. But what is enjoyment? It is quality of life, ultimately. And if we look soberly at that concept, it means a pain-free and content life for us and our relatives. To have enough to eat, to be healthy, to have a roof over our head and the feeling of safety and security in a circle of beloved people, and a meaningful task, a job we like.

The insight that what seems normal is an illusion may help us to stay lively and consciously walk-through life with a lively heart, a feeling heart. We are born anew with every heartbeat. One day it will be our last. Before the silence. But maybe we will go on again. Maybe the silence was merely a pause, and only afterward can we really appreciate the gift of life.

14

CURIOSITY FOR THE NEW NORMAL

At the end of rehab, we don't know for sure if we have truly mastered the crisis – after all, the big test at home is still ahead of us. But we have come the better part of the way, and things look good if we paced ourselves well and developed a plan for the future, and if everyone is on board. It is comparable to an insolvency: at the start no one was sure if things could continue, total collapse was imminent – but now, a way out of the crisis has been found, and things can continue, maybe even better than before.

The patients return home, but they do not return to their old normal. Too many things have changed. The sooner they accept that, and the better they manage to embrace it and even look forward to it, the more they will be able to enjoy their new quality of life. And not only smart minds should be able to do that, but as many people as possible.

I want to get to the point where we – every one of us and society in general – speak about the evolution of a crisis, so that we are prepared. And I want to demonstrate that there are always alternatives. I could fill pages and pages with stories of how my patients changed their lives "afterwards". It isn't that life changed – *they* changed *it*. That is a crucial difference. Am I the victim or the designer of my life? With our foundation, we want to enable people to act as designers. You will find some stories on the internet, on the *Stilgezet* homepage. Every now and then I was allowed to be a "godfather" to a new phase of life, when patients told me about the pain, they felt about no longer being able to do certain things. "Have you ever thought of…", I asked. At first, I often heard "No, that's not for me", or even brusque rejection. But a day or a week later their resistance had softened a little, and things were progressing step by step. They made adjustments to an alternative we had offered, so that now it would suit them. The former professional swimmer now coaches the young talent and is enthusiastic: "I used to swim up and down by myself for hours. It meant everything to me. Now I still swim, but no longer for hours. Instead, I stand on the pool edge for hours, walking up and down, and my heart overflows sometimes when I see the progress of my little ones." There was water gleaming in his eyes, too, probably because of too much chlorine in the air.

I remember numerous executives, people who identified with their work completely and who learned from their illness that there is a life beside their job. Once a former patient confided in me: "There are times when I become melancholy when I think how much time I spent in the office. The many meaningful things I could have done!" She paused and then said something I had heard a few times from people who had left a crisis behind: "Ultimately, I'm grateful. Without my illness I just would have gone on like that. How much I would have missed."

Yes indeed, one can miss life's intensity – but the normal does not just fall in your lap either, you have to work for it. Step by step, different circumstances must be considered. Now, we are working on programs for all transitional phases in our foundation *Stilgezet*, to enable patients to really find their way to their new normal.

What happens, we ask, when a patient gets stuck in an in-between, so to speak, between the old normal which they see as the Promised Land, and a new normal which they do not want to accept? It is sad when people get in their own way on the road to their new normal, out if the crisis, steadily upwards. On the other hand, I am also sure that if everyone involved does their job well at the key points of the graph (see above at the end of the chapter OPENING), the patients will have a higher quality of life than before in the end, even though they may experience physical limitations. I don't want to trivialize anything, but the decades of my experience with people who fell out of their familiar normal have shown me that quality of life will increase for the simple reason alone that one has learned to be grateful to still be here. Life turned out to be so fragile, such a great miracle – and isn't it the greatest miracle that I'm still here?

This great miracle makes it relatively easy to bear the fact that one cannot or should not ride one's bike for thirty kilometers, but only twenty – and that one should take things more slowly and yes, do without some of them when one's new self turns out to be less physically robust than one's old one. It can, however, be the other way around as well, particularly with illnesses which caused insufficient oxygen supply by the heart's diminished pumping performance. A leaking heart valve at an advanced stage leads to a dilation of the heart, the enlargement of a heart chamber – which diminished the patient's capability considerably: they will be out of breath from the slightest exertion, they need to pause when climbing stairs, and the color of their face tends to be blueish to purple.

Once the heart's pumping power is restored, oxygen saturation will increase. Such patients beam at me after the operation, hardly able to believe it: "I feel reborn, Doc! I can breathe properly again!" Some patients call me Doc. I like that. The trust of my patients means the world to me, and I feel how it warms my heart.

Patients whose physical abilities are limited after a severe intervention often speak of their new life, too. Some say: "I escaped from the jaws of death."

If you have mastered a crisis, you have achieved something big. You have a future again, even if it may look different from what you imagined. There were times during the crisis when it wasn't thinkable that there could even be a future. And there were times when you hoped it would be the old future – until you realized that that is gone forever. Yet this loss is nothing painful, but a reward which suggests I've made it!

We can only properly "make it" if everyone goes along with it, if relatives and friends and colleagues and neighbors – in short, everyone around us – understand that it is normal for the normal to change. There is no point in resisting.

Then when a neighbor or relative or colleague one day faces a similar situation, they are not alone. We can switch on a light for them, tell them the coordinates, to help them find their new normal. We can be a role model for others and in this fashion pave the way for them through what we do and don't do. We are not afraid to mention taboo subjects. We are not stressed by it; the relatives might be, but we can help and tell them what is important now. We can do a lot of good when we have mastered a crisis well.

When I visited my parents recently, we looked at photos. My father is in his nineties now, got a new hip in 2020 and survived a COVID infection, and in 2021 got two new knees and a pacemaker (the latter not inserted by me, even though I would have liked to do it, but I was too far away when he needed it). Anyway, we were looking at photos, and there was this one picture with the greenhouses. Suddenly I was a boy of twelve or thirteen again. Back then we harvested two-hundred and fifty tons of tomatoes every year, and all the children helped. But we also got up to a lot of mischief. When I look back, I remember a very nice childhood. And I was an enthusiastic observer. Everything interested me, and I would pester my parents and older siblings with questions. Why is this so? Today it is my father who sometimes asks me: "Why is this so?"

Once I answered: "Because the ant crawled in a circle." I saw it before me like back then, when it crawled along a strangely arc-shaped cucumber in one of the greenhouses. Up and down the ant crawled. Decades later, when I had already created the crisis graph which

I introduced at the beginning of this book, this ant suddenly came to my mind. And it seemed to me that what today is the matter closest to my heart laid its first track back then.

The small ant trail has become a path. I very much hope that it will turn into a wide road, leading to many people's hearts. Have I reached your heart? Do you have a story you wish to share? Write to us on the homepage of our foundation. I am looking forward to it.

All the best for you!

Yours,

Ehsan Natour

ACKNOWLEDGMENTS

The journey on my personal "life graph" began when I was nineteen, when I left my comfort zone and arrived in Europe where I was a complete stranger. I want to express my deepest gratitude to my parents and siblings here for their support along my path.

I am much obliged to my patients and their relatives for sharing their misfortunes and life experience, and especially for entrusting their hearts to me.

A big thank-you goes to the many nurses. They are always there for our patients, accompany us doctors on our assignments and do amazing work. They listen, they care and have their eyes open day and night. In my profession you don't go very far without your team, and thus I want to mention my colleagues here from whom I was able to learn many things.

I explicitly want to thank the Scorpio Europa Verlag. With their support, the book *When Life Stands Still* will find a good home amongst the readers.

My special thanks go to the excellent writer Shirley Michaela Seul who was convinced after a thirty-minute phone conversation that the world needs this book.

I robbed my dear family of many hours and days during the completion of this book. I thank you for your patience and your love.

A heart-felt thanks also goes to you, dear readers.

And finally, a significant thank-you is appropriate for my best friend who permanently challenges me, who is my partner as well as my opponent, who makes me think and motivates me to continue to improve myself...my best friend, the heart.

SOURCES AND FURTHER READING

Barwich, A.S.: Smellosophy. What the Nose Tells the Mind. Cambridge, Mass: Harvard University Press 2020

Friedl, Reinhard: The Source of all Things. A Heart Surgeon's Quest to Understand Our Most Mysterious Organ. New York: St. Martin's Press 2021

Gilbert, Avery: What the Nose Knows. The Science of Scent in Everyday Life. New York: Crown Publishing Group 2008

Maio, Giovanne: *Den kranken Menschen verstehen: für eine Medizin der Zuwendung.* [Understanding the Sick Human Being: for a Medicine of Loving Care] Freiburg: Herder 2020 (new edition)

Pause, Bettina M.: *Alles Geruchssache: wie unsere Nase steuert was wir wollen und wen wir lieben* [It's All a Matter of Smell: How Our Nose Decides What We Want and Whom We Love]. Munich: Piper 2020

Peipe, Kurt: *Dem Leben auf den Fersen. Zu Fuß von Flensburg nach Rom – die Geschichte meiner Reise zu mir selbst.* [On the Heels of Life. Walking from Flensburg to Rome – the Story of the Journey to Myself]. Munich: Droemer 2008

Schneider, Oliver: *Der Wille entscheidet: Krisen bewältigen, Verhandlunge gewinnen* [The Will Decides: Managing Crises, Winning Negotiations] Munich: Ariston 2021

Vanbuskirk, David J.: My Life with Death. The Firsthand Account of an Undertaker. Denver: Outskirts Press 2014

STICHTING STILGEZET

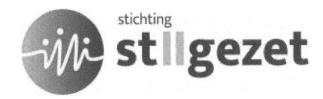

Most people are afraid of the unknown. When something bad happens, we crave familiarity and normality. We leave our comfort zone only unwillingly, and we are not well practiced in living outside what we are used to. There is no one-size-fits-all solution to process the confusion and fears which can arise when life "comes to a standstill". Everyone reacts and handles such a situation differently. It may concern a life crisis, a separation, a stock market crash or an illness.

Many people around the world experience a serious and sometimes life-saving medical treatment. Suddenly, life appears to "come to a standstill" – and not only the patient's life, but also the lives of their families and friends. The doctors and nurses, too, are affected. This standstill of life is a dramatic experience. People often decide consciously or unconsciously not to deal with it too much. But it is of vital importance to come to terms with the time of the standstill, not least for the healing process and "life afterwards".

Stichting Stilgezet, a foundation born in the Netherlands, provides answers, based not only on medicine but also other means of expression. The book "When Life Stands Still" by Dr. Ehsan Natour is part of this as well as a play, a musical composition, and many other tools. In this way, the indescribable becomes palpable. *Stichting Stilgezet* fills the gap left by science, which those affected often experience as a place of fear. Artistic "translation" helps to illustrate and eventually integrate dramatic experiences and confusing emotions – topics such as death, fear, anger, and grief. And of course, art offers comfort and understanding where reason and high-tech medicine fall short. Most importantly, it promotes the positive feeling: you are not alone.

Stichting Stilgezet works closely with scientific research to understand and clarify the emotional and social context of this significant phase of life. We offer help and support for all those affected by a crisis situation, as well as orientation for medical professionals.

www.stilgezet.nl